Cooperative Crisis Management and Avian Influenza

A Risk Assessment Guide for International Contagious Disease Prevention and Risk Mitigation

Donald F. Thompson and Renata P. Louie

Center for Technology and National Security Policy

March 2006

Colonel Donald F. Thompson is a senior research fellow in the Center for Technology and National Security Policy at the National Defense University. He is a Senior Flight Surgeon in the United States Air Force and specializes in family medicine and preventive medicine. Dr. Thompson can be contacted at donald.thompson@af.mil.

Captain Renata P. Louie, U.S. Navy, is a senior military fellow in the Institute for National Strategic Studies at the National Defense University. She is an East Asia regional specialist with special focus on China and Japan. Her research interests include international negotiations, conflict/crisis management, and nontraditional security challenges. CAPT Louie can be contacted at louier@ndu.edu or (202) 685-3839.

Defense & Technology Papers *are published by the National Defense University Center for Technology and National Security Policy, Fort Lesley J. McNair, Washington, DC. CTNSP publications are available online at http://www.ndu.edu/ctnsp/publications.html.*

Contents

Executive Summary

The nature of infectious disease outbreaks and their potential for rapid global spread require enhanced preparedness, including a fine-tuned ability to communicate, cooperate, and collaborate, within countries and across international borders on very short notice and with minimal bureaucratic delay. Cooperation must be predicated upon a clear understanding of national and international roles and responsibilities at all phases of a crisis. The importance of communication, collaboration, and cooperation cannot be overemphasized.

The lack of diagnostic tools to evaluate preparedness or identify weaknesses of individual countries creates a dangerous vulnerability to understanding roles and responsibilities and enhancing international cooperation. In its 2005 *Responding to the Avian Influenza Pandemic Threat: Recommended Strategic Actions*, the World Health Organization acknowledged the lack of a "regional or global tool for evaluating the actual status of preparedness in individual countries and pinpointing weaknesses that need to be addressed." Whether dealing with countries that are developing or developed, large or small, "governments that fail to prepare for [such] disasters are preparing to fail." The hurricanes on the Gulf Coast of the United States in 2005 demonstrate this point fully and have renewed awareness of the importance of deliberative preparedness planning at all levels of government and the private sector.

This paper proposes a risk assessment and mitigation strategy designed to give both national authorities and international organizations the diagnostic tool needed to evaluate preparedness, identify country-level weaknesses, and prioritize scarce resources to combat avian influenza. This tool could help authorities and agencies at all levels of government identify risk factors and actions that may be taken to reduce vulnerabilities to communicable disease outbreaks; prevent animal-to-human disease transmission; improve the response to a communicable disease outbreak; and empower government authorities to communicate with local, national, and international partners. Without adequate prevention efforts, a communicable disease outbreak can rapidly spread and develop into an epidemic. Without an adequate response plan, an epidemic is more likely to become a pandemic. The prevention and response phases of crisis management are aimed at the most important element of cooperative crisis management: preventing loss of life. Senior decisionmakers who must make crisis management choices in the face of limited information often need practical experience to support this process. The risk assessment and mitigation strategy becomes an essential tool to which these decisionmakers may turn in a crisis.

An effective response requires rapid, coordinated action by all involved local, regional, and central government agencies with clear roles and responsibilities so time and effort are not wasted. Infectious diseases and migratory birds that carry some of these diseases do not recognize national borders, so information-sharing is critical both within a country and between states and within multilateral organizations that support their members at the international level. One of the fading lessons from the SARS epidemic is that the nature of infectious disease outbreaks dictates that every hour counts. Decisionmakers must act promptly to reduce further spread of a contagion while simultaneously taking steps to identify and characterize the threat and communicate with others who must take similar actions. This tool facilitates that process.

If information is withheld, other countries may find it necessary to take actions to protect their own citizens and interests. Such actions may or may not be warranted, and more draconian measures by nonaffected countries could have serious consequences at all levels—national, regional, and global. This tool focuses on the critical elements of prevention and response to a communicable disease outbreak, and provides the common language for both domestic and international cooperation, collaboration and communication.

This risk assessment and mitigation strategy tool was developed to meet the following objectives:

- to lay the foundation for development of an international standard for communicable disease prevention and response;

- to educate authorities and agencies on factors important to preventing and responding to an outbreak;

- to assist those who might benefit from greater insight regarding crisis management and prevention in the context of, but not limited to, public health crises;

- to respond to the need for greater collaboration and integration of veterinary and medical disciplines in both prevention and response efforts regarding avian influenza and other communicable diseases so as to strengthen, not weaken, the impact that animal and human surveillance and detection systems can offer ;

- to encourage international collaboration and openness by demonstrating that risk mitigation does not always have to be expensive but the economic impact and implications of lack of openness could be extremely costly for humanity.

The value of this risk assessment methodology lies in its practicality. The case study demonstrates how the tool can be used. Senior government decisionmakers, as well as village, town, city, state, provincial, national, and other public health and veterinary health officials should consider this tool as a roadmap for preventive action and response. It will serve as a guide for communicating within and across government bureaucracies, for educating the public on measures that will mitigate the dangers posed by communicable disease outbreaks, and for informing the media so that it may play a more proactive role both before and during a crisis. Finally, this tool will serve organizations such as the World Health Organization, Food and Agricultural Organization, World Organisation for Animal Health and potential donors and others responsible for prioritizing interventions at the global level.

The assessment process described in this paper allows users to become familiar with the risk factors associated with avian influenza and to take initial steps in self-assessment and disease transmission risk reduction. Worksheets are provided so users can conduct their own assessments. The steps in this process are:

- *Step 1—Local Self-Assessment*. This step identifies in great detail the widely recognized risk factors (ecological, infrastructure, and response) that contribute to disease transmission risk. Users may utilize these factors to identify areas in their own specific environment where mitigation efforts should be focused to improve preparedness as efficiently as possible.

- *Step 2—External Perceptions*. This step considers external perceptions of a country's internal preparedness and response capabilities. Here, transparency factors are applied to the self-assessment process because they are important aspects of managing external perceptions. External perceptions can cause unaffected countries to consider more drastic measures for self-protection. This step lays the foundation for better understanding contradictions between external and internal perceptions of an affected country's preparedness and helps identify areas where communication, cooperation, and collaboration can take place.

- *Step 3—International Response*. This step represents a blending of the transmission characteristics of the disease agent (avian influenza) and the likelihood of interrupting disease transmission in a particular geographic area. This step allows determination of the transmission risk for a specific disease by country and locality, taking into account the WHO Pandemic Alert Phases for avian influenza.

- *Step 4—Identify Areas for Intervention*. Based on the cumulative scores obtained in Steps 1 through 3, users can now seek opportunities for intervention (risk reduction). The careful deliberation about potential courses of action before a crisis occurs allows steps to be identified that, while serious and not without consequence, may be more effective than draconian steps that might be considered and implemented in the heat of the moment when pressure to respond may lead to actions that may not be completely thought through.

- *Step 5—Take Action*. This step points to the actual mitigation measures that can be taken to decrease the risk of infectious disease transmission.

- *Step 6—Repeat Self-Assessment to Determine Effect of Interventions*. This final step allows users to determine whether intervention efforts were adequate to decrease the level of risk sufficiently.

4

Section One
Introduction

On December 26, 2004, the international community awoke to an unthinkable catastrophe: a tsunami that devastated parts of South and Southeast Asia with untold cost in human life. While the international response was impressive, debate immediately ensued as to whether such destruction and human loss could have been mitigated in part through an early warning system and better national and international planning and preparedness. Hurricane Katrina, and its effects on the Gulf Coast of the United States in general and the city of New Orleans in particular, demonstrated that even a technologically advanced country like the United States, with a sophisticated system for warning of hazardous weather and massive disaster management infrastructure and considerable expertise, was not prepared for a scenario many deemed possible, but most thought unimaginable. The failures in connection with Katrina appear to be largely a result of inadequate planning and preparedness.

An avian influenza pandemic is a crisis looming. The U.S. Secretary for Health and Human Services, in his remarks at the convening of the States on Pandemic Influenza Preparedness in December 2005, stated that, "When it comes to a pandemic we are overdue and under prepared."[1] Indeed, the international community is overdue and under prepared for another global pandemic. The worldwide influenza pandemic of 1918 should serve as a frightening harbinger for the international community to better prepare and plan for the possibility of a repeat event, yet many countries are paralyzed by the enormity of such a task in the face of other more immediate demands. To some, the 1918 influenza pandemic seems like ancient history, so when comparisons are made between the devastation almost a century ago to potential outcomes today, the sheer number of deaths and the impact on regional and global security become unthinkable.

Planning and preparing for such a pandemic becomes a larger-than-life task, and the international community runs the risk of denying that anything can be done to protect from what would certainly be a doomsday scenario. In the context of competing demands and a false belief that higher priority equals higher risk, authorities often devote all their preparations to the worst possible outcome of such a pandemic, overlooking preventive action that will provide real risk reduction. If preparedness paralyzes, prevention barely lights up on the radar scope. In today's world of competing crises, it is easy to compartmentalize complex problems: take them out, debate them, and put them away because the problems are seemingly too difficult to address.

> **...authorities often devote all their preparations to the worst possible outcome of such a pandemic, overlooking preventive action that will provide real risk reduction.**

---

[1] Michael Leavitt, "Remarks to the Convening of the States on Pandemic Influenza Preparedness," December 5, 2005. Available at: <http://www.hhs.gov/news/speech/2005/051205.html>, accessed February 4, 2006.

They are taken back out only when the crisis hits, but by then it is too late to take risk reduction steps.

One of the already fading lessons from the severe acute respiratory syndrome (SARS) epidemic is that the nature of infectious disease outbreaks dictates that "every hour counts."[2] Decisionmakers must act promptly to reduce further spread of contagion while they simultaneously identify and characterize the threat and communicate with others who must take similar actions. This means that the transition from pre-outbreak to outbreak to epidemic to pandemic may occur almost imperceptibly and make the initial steps along the continuum toward crisis response a daily reality. The human tendency to compartmentalize complex problems in the face of more pressing demands and the nature of infectious disease outbreaks, which require early detection and rapid response "as the window of opportunity for preventing deaths and further spread closes quickly,"[3] threaten to bring out the worst aspects of the state of international preparedness: little communication, poor cooperation, and ineffective collaboration in the face of an unthinkable international threat.

Creating an Assessment Tool

The importance of communication, collaboration, and cooperation to bridge gaps cannot be overemphasized. Because of the potential for rapid global spread of an infectious outbreak, preparedness mandates a fine-tuned ability to interact both vertically and horizontally, within a state and across borders, on very short order. This means that the appropriate communications infrastructure and processes must be operational and regularly exercised, assessed, and improved; a framework of interagency and international cooperation must be in place and all potential participants must be comfortable with its procedures well before a crisis occurs. Cooperation cannot occur in a vacuum. It must be predicated upon a clear understanding of national and international roles and responsibilities at all phases of a crisis and open acknowledgement of the international consequences of inaction.

The lack of diagnostic tools to evaluate preparedness or identify weaknesses at the country level has been a challenge both to understanding roles and responsibilities and to enhancing international cooperation. In 2005, the World Health Organization (WHO) published several important strategy papers. In particular, the *WHO Global Influenza Preparedness Plan* outlines the organization's role and makes recommendations for national measures before and during pandemics. It defines WHO and national objectives as well as actions.

---

[2] Christine Loh and Civic Exchange, eds, *At the Epicentre: Hong Kong and the SARS Outbreak* (Hong Kong: Hong Kong University Press, 2004), 238.
[3] Ibid.

It does not provide a "regional or global tool for evaluating the actual status of preparedness in individual countries and pinpointing weaknesses that need to be addressed,"[4]a shortfall that the WHO acknowledged in another recent document, *Responding to the Avian Influenza Pandemic Threat: Recommended Strategic Actions*. It also emphasizes national pandemic preparedness planning. But if delaying or averting a pandemic is the goal, then prevention needs to be confronted aggressively and proactively.

A Global Strategy for the Progressive Control of Highly Pathogenic Avian Influenza, produced by the Food and Agriculture Organization (FAO, Rome) and World Organisation for Animal Health (*Office International des Epizooties* [OIE], Paris) in collaboration with the WHO (Geneva) tackles prevention issues, providing "a vision and goal towards diminishing the risk of avian influenza to humans and poultry" along with "approaches and implementation plans for the control of avian influenza." The risk assessment and mitigation strategy tool advanced in this paper goes extends the WHO, FAO and OIE vision by enabling users to operationalize that vision and quantify progress.

In the United States, both the *National Strategy for Pandemic Influenza* and the U.S. Department of Health and Human Services *HHS Pandemic Influenza Plan* focus primarily on the response aspect of an avian influenza pandemic.[5] Although the *National Strategy for Pandemic Influenza* stresses the need for surveillance and detection, both avian and human, it does not emphasize the need for a multidisciplinary approach with close cooperation between veterinary and medical experts for "understanding and developing the multiple links between these two fields…essential for establishing effective surveillance, preparedness, and response strategies and for developing appropriate, government-wide mechanisms for risk assessment and management."[6] This paper underscores the need for greater collaboration between veterinary and medical professions and provides a framework for risk assessment and management in the context of both prevention and response.

The risk assessment and mitigation tool advanced in this paper responds to the need for both a regional/global tool to evaluate the status of preparedness of individual countries and a more cooperative connection among regions. This preventive action tool creates a scientifically sound strategy for risk assessment and mitigation and serves several objectives. First, it lays the foundation for development of an international standard for

---

[4] World Health Organization, "Responding to the avian influenza pandemic threat: Recommended strategic actions." Available at:
<http://www.who.int/csr/resources/publications/influenza/WHO_CDS_CSR_GIP_2005_8/en/>, accessed October 23, 2005, 16.
[5] The *National Strategy for Pandemic Influenza* of November 2005 by the Homeland Security Council is available at: <http://www.whitehouse.gov/homeland/pandemic-influenza.html>, accessed October 23, 2005. The *HHS Pandemic Influenza Plan*, November 2005 is available at:
<http://www.hhs.gov/pandemicflu/plan/, accessed October 23, 2005>.
[6] Liam Donaldson and Debby Reynolds, "UK government collaborations to manage threats to animal and human health," *British Medicine Journal* 331, no, 5, November 26, 2005, 1216.

communicable disease prevention and response. This is vital if communication, cooperation, and collaboration are to occur both within countries and across international borders. Infectious disease pathogens, like avian influenza, do not recognize borders.

Second, this tool serves a teaching function. It can educate authorities and agencies at all levels of government on factors important to preventing disease transmission, responses to a communicable disease outbreak, and the importance of information-sharing at the international level. It includes practical strategies and tools that will be useful in developing information-sharing procedures within and between countries.

Third, and more broadly, this risk assessment and mitigation tool can assist local, city, state, provincial, national or federal authorities, and many other users, such as public and private researchers, analysts, and the media, who might gain greater insight regarding crisis management and prevention in the context of not only public health emergencies, but also natural disasters and even terrorism. This knowledge will foster cooperation among these disparate sectors; reduce the likelihood of inaccurate media reports and unreasonable response expectations; and improve the efforts of scientific, policy, and risk communication researchers.

Fourth, this tool will encourage international collaboration and transparency by demonstrating that risk mitigation does not always have to be expensive and that the economic impact and implications of a lack of transparency justify a serious reexamination of international consequences in today's interconnected global economy.

> *...perception is reality for many... Lack of information...sometimes drives political decisionmakers to take actions that ultimately may not effectively counter the threat and can...negatively impact political and economic stability.*

Finally, perception is reality for many people. National leaders who are unaware of what other countries are doing to mitigate and respond to the risks of communicable diseases are forced to speculate about the danger posed to their own countries by the actions (or non-actions) of others. Lack of information often forces governments to elevate perceived risk and sometimes drives political decisionmakers to take actions that ultimately may not effectively counter the threat and can result in secondary and tertiary effects that negatively impact political and economic stability. This risk assessment methodology connects the world in a way that helps decisionmakers both identify areas for local improvement and determine whether additional protective measures should be taken within one's own borders if lack of information about an affected country instills uncertainty.

Key Assumptions

This study is built upon several assumptions for mitigating an international contagious disease epidemic, particularly an avian influenza pandemic. First, it assumes that a coordinated international response to a disease outbreak is possible, despite diverse languages, cultures, geography, populations, demographics, and resources. These differences among individual citizens, ethnic groups, regions, and nation-states make for many communication and coordination challenges, but cooperative crisis management is achievable in the near term. It requires, as a starting point, common terms of reference, vocabulary, roles and responsibilities, and a common understanding of goals.

Second, self-assessment of disease transmission risks is possible. Identifying risk factors and assigning weights to the level of risk a country faces help the affected country identify and prioritize areas for mitigation and preventive action and provides direction for multilateral organizations and donor states. Findings can be communicated both vertically and horizontally, helping government agencies in the cooperation and collaboration process within jurisdictions and political boundaries and with external actors.

Third, self-assessment results and external assessment of disease transmission risks associated with a specific geographic location may differ. Concerns and misperceptions can arise from such contradictions. In fact, however, the mere existence of differences in perception regarding another party's self-assessment can be helpful in a number of ways. First, cooperation results from relationships among people. The opportunity to discuss these differences creates the environment in which the kind of cooperative relationships between governments can be formed so they can pursue mutually supportive strategic risk assessment and management. Second, such dialogue helps actors focus on common interests and concerns while providing an environment in which both sides can question their own assumptions and move toward constructing a more effective strategy to reduce risk. Third, dialogue about differences, if properly channeled, can lead to the generation of new ideas and the design of a risk reduction strategy that works for all concerned—in a more comprehensive way that takes into account that infectious diseases like avian influenza are global problems and cannot be dealt with simply at the national level.

Fourth, many mitigation opportunities exist, but local conditions determine which ones are practical. Infrastructure, resource limitations, and competing priorities all impact the relative order in which actions will be taken. Local authorities will determine these priorities, bearing in mind both internal and external consequences of their actions and inactions.

Finally, increasing transparency about local conditions is likely to reduce misunderstanding and miscommunication. Inaccurate assumptions about intentions are often made in countries where cultural understanding may be incomplete. Increased communication using a common communicable disease control lexicon will reduce the likelihood of serious international missteps that may be taken during an international crisis response.

Purpose of Study

The purpose of this paper is to bridge the major gap identified by the WHO—the lack of a "regional or global tool for evaluating the actual status of preparedness in individual countries and pinpointing weaknesses that need to be addressed."[7] This paper provides authorities and agencies at all levels within governments and international organizations a risk assessment and mitigation tool that will identify risk factors and actions that may be taken to reduce susceptibility to communicable disease outbreaks; prevent animal-to-human disease transmission; assist in responding to a communicable disease outbreak; empower government authorities to communicate with local, national, and international partners; and ultimately help prioritize needs and intervention efforts more effectively at the national, regional and global level.

At the global level, this tool is intended to offer international organizations, such as the World Health Organization, Food and Agricultural Organization, International Organization for Animal Health, World Bank, International Monetary Fund, nongovernmental organizations, and private foundations a systematic way to prioritize interventions. The potential international benefits are obvious: prioritizing needs helps identify high-risk countries and opportunities for preventive intervention as well as identifying the minimal crisis management steps for protection of human and animal life at the local level that could have enormous impact globally.

Village, town, city, state, provincial, or other public health and veterinary health officials will consider this tool as a useful roadmap for preventive action and response. This tool is intended to serve as a guide for communicating within and across government bureaucracies, to educate the public on measures that will mitigate the dangers posed by communicable disease outbreaks, and to inform the media so that it may play a more proactive role both before and during a crisis.

Organization of Paper

This paper presents the results of a research effort to build a risk assessment and mitigation strategy for international contagious disease prevention. It addresses the connection between local self-assessment, the international community's perception of a country's efforts to prevent or respond to a communicable disease outbreak, and a methodology for developing a risk assessment and mitigation strategy for avian influenza. In short, it attempts to provide the international community with a framework for implementing an effective international strategy of prevention and response. The paper is organized as follows:

- Section 1 places the prevention of an influenza pandemic in the context of crisis planning and preparedness and highlights the importance of international communication, collaboration, and cooperation to preparedness efforts. It underscores the current lack of a regional/global assessment tool and the linkages required for improved communication, collaboration, and cooperation both domestically and internationally.

---

[7] Ibid.

- Section 2 develops working definitions of the elements that constitute the underpinnings of cooperative crisis management. It distinguishes disasters from crises. It also defines tipping points between pre-crisis and crisis events and details two phases associated with crisis management—response and prevention.

- Section 3 identifies the five risk factor areas that must be assessed to identify mitigation opportunities. They include: ecological, infrastructure, response, transparency, and disease-specific outbreak and transmission factors.

- Section 4 describes disease transmission risk zones and proposes a methodology to assess the risk of an avian influenza outbreak. It also links the assessment tool to outbreak factors published by the WHO.

- Section 5 studies the current global situation with avian influenza to demonstrate how the risk assessment tool can be utilized at local, national, and international levels to reduce risk, improve preparedness, and facilitate cooperation in an international crisis.

- Section 6 summarizes how this risk assessment tool can help lay the foundation for a regional cooperation mechanism and suggests possible future methods for building on academic disaster response tools developed in the past.

Section Two
Crisis Management and Crisis Phases

Disasters of all types have led to the loss of millions of lives in the past quarter-century. *Natural disasters* have ranged from sudden cataclysmic weather phenomena—tornados, hurricanes, earthquakes, tsunamis, and wildfires—to extremes of temperature and rainfall with resulting droughts or floods. *Manmade disasters* include human conflict up to and including full-scale war, industrial accidents, or widespread environmental destruction. The disruption of the normal lives of an affected population measures the true impact of a disaster. Infrastructure may be totally disrupted, requiring extensive time to reestablish normal function. Recovery efforts may last years, and local conditions may never be restored to their pre-disaster state. Because disasters are generally considered "low probability/high impact" events, responsible authorities sometimes defer funding for disaster planning efforts in lieu of current tasks and projects that seem to justify immediate action and attention.[8]

The WHO defines a *disaster* as "a sudden ecological phenomenon of sufficient magnitude to require external assistance."[9] In the public health setting, it might be described as when "the number of casualties exceeds the ability of the medical infrastructure to provide care without external assistance."[10] Others define disasters as an imbalance in the availability of medical care and a maldistribution of medical resources versus casualties within a community.[11] In all definitions, disasters are something outside the normal experience of daily life that requires a change in one's perspective from daily management style and thinking. World War II correspondent Ernie Pyle described this shift in perspective when he observed that to the individual soldier, the war was rarely bigger than 100 yards on either side. In disaster and crisis management, while one must be skilled in his or her 100 yards of a disaster, he or she needs a larger view to significantly impact disaster planning and response.[12]

In contrast, a *crisis* takes place when a serious breakdown occurs in a system's ability to cope with a situation, resulting in further escalation or spread of the negative effects that prompted the initial response.[13] Such disruption may be the intentional outcome of a terrorist attack, the goals of which often are the intentional disruption of the usual elements of power in society (finance, communication, justice), the public's alienation from the government because of doubts about leadership competence, and the breakup of

---

[8] David E. Hogan and Jonathan L. Burnstein, "Basic Physics of Disasters," in David E. Hogan and Jonathan L. Burnstein, eds., *Disaster Medicine* (Baltimore: Lippincott, Williams, and Wilkins, 2002), 3.
[9] Eric Noji, *The Public Health Consequences of Disasters* (New York: Oxford University Press, 1997).
[10] Hogan and Bernstein, 3.
[11] Ibid., 4.
[12] Ibid., 4.
[13] Ian Mitroff states that a major crisis results when there is a serious breakdown or malfunction between people, organizations, and technologies inasmuch as it invalidates critical assumptions that people, organizations, and societies had been making about people, organizations, and technologies. Ian I. Mitroff, *Crisis Leadership: Planning for the Unthinkable* (Hoboken, NJ: John Wiley and Sons, Inc., 2004).

international partnerships and coalitions. Similar consequences often occur when the crisis results from a natural disaster such as a flood, tsunami, earthquake, or hurricane, since the public focuses on basic survival needs. When the system is incapable of providing food, water, and housing in the face of a devastating loss of infrastructure, governmental authorities are often blamed for these failures.

Public health crises such as SARS or avian influenza can disrupt civil society even more than a natural disaster or an intentional terrorist act. The public perceives that the health care delivery system and public health agencies exist to provide adequate protection from such illnesses and are able to effectively treat cases that develop. When an infectious disease outbreak occurs despite the government's seemingly best efforts at prevention and treatment, public confidence is often shaken to the core as people begin to question their own safety. The presence of functioning finance, communications, and justice systems is not sufficiently reassuring when a mysterious disease strikes for unknown reasons.

In the field of epidemiology and disease control, a *disease outbreak* is a large number of cases of a disease that occur in a short period of time. An *epidemic* is determined to exist after an investigation of the disease outbreak confirms that excessive cases do, in fact, exist based on a specific case definition and the background numbers of cases expected in the particular area in a defined period of time. A *pandemic* is an epidemic that is widespread across a country, continent, or a large population, possibly worldwide.

When the system designed to deal with the outbreak of an infectious disease fails to detect it or to keep it from spreading (that is, it becomes an epidemic, or worse, a pandemic) and its spread can no longer be controlled, then a crisis has occurred. The public quickly develops doubts about the competency of government officials, since the general assumption is that public health systems should be sufficient to provide protection. Government officials often respond defensively, which deepens public doubts and leads to accusations of subterfuge and malicious intent. Increasing public and media attention to every response detail causes officials to carefully consider each action before it is taken, slowing the response and limiting actions to those that are most defensible in the public eye. Government credibility is greatly compromised by this behavior, transparency is reduced in response to external criticism, and the destructive vicious cycle continues.

Such were the findings of several governmental review panels that evaluated the public sector's handling of the SARS outbreak in Hong Kong in 2003. Two reports pointed to a lack of leadership, absence of a strategy and contingency planning, and poor communication and crisis management skills as major weaknesses of the healthcare system.[14] The fact that no one with the power to make decisions was responsible for error did little to address public demands for increased accountability and transparency on the part of the authorities.[15]

Similar outcomes were seen in the muddled government response to Hurricane Katrina on the U.S. Gulf Coast in 2005. Local disaster and hurricane evacuation plans had been developed yet were not executed by local officials. Alternative steps were quickly taken in an attempt to care for displaced residents as flooding made the city of New Orleans uninhabitable, but the full scope of resource requirements had not been considered, response efforts failed, and a crisis quickly developed. Decisionmakers at all levels of government appeared paralyzed as criticism mounted, news reports about the degree of suffering were embellished, and confidence in government officials who were seemingly unable to manage the crisis plummeted.

Crisis Management

Crisis management involves "a process of strategic planning for a crisis or negative turning point, a process that removes some of the risk and uncertainty from the negative occurrence and thereby allows the organization to be in greater control of its own destiny."[16] A *tipping point* is the moment in time where a crucial decision must be made. Such decisions may include immediate response steps, measures to collect additional information about the scope of an incident, notification of other agencies and authorities who may need to be involved in preventing enlargement of the crisis, and communication with the public about steps to take to protect from further harm.

When correct tipping point decisions are made, the system's ability to respond to the event is maintained or enhanced. When an incorrect tipping point decision is made, or when no decision is made, the system's response is degraded, public trust is reduced, and more effort must be made simply to maintain the system's integrity. As incorrect or inadequate decisions continue to be made and actions are insufficient to provide support to the system, risk and uncertainties increase until the system ultimately fails.

Identifying tipping points by assessing potential crisis situations and developing comprehensive, coordinated plans for prevention and response can remove much of the risk and uncertainty inherent in a potential crisis scenario. Decisionmakers can then explore the likely outcomes of various courses of action, including the second- and third-

---

[14]For detailed information see the following two reports: SARS Expert Committee, "SARS in Hong Kong: From Experience to Action," October 2, 2003. Available at < http://www.sars-expertcom.gov hk/english/reports/reports html>, accessed December 7, 2005; and Hong Kong Hospital Authority, "Report of the Hospital Authority Review Panel on the SARS Outbreak (September 2003) and Hospital Authority's Response," October 16, 2003. Available at <http://www.ha.org hk/sars/ps/report/reviewpanel_e.pdf>, accessed December 7, 2005.

[15] Loh and Civic Exchange, eds., xiii.

[16] Chris Skinner and Gary Mersham, *Disaster Management: A Guide to Issues Management and Crisis Communication* (Oxford: Oxford University Press, 2002), 23.

level unintended consequences.[17] These crucial steps will be demonstrated here in the case of an infectious disease outbreak of avian influenza, and its potential deterioration into an epidemic or worldwide pandemic as widespread human-to-human transmission develops (Section 5).

Openness about the contents of prevention and response plans and the degree of local preparedness gives the public and the media a valuable perspective on the degree of vulnerability and the steps that must be taken to effectively respond to a crisis. This openness also informs the public on roles and responsibilities of government and steps that the general public itself should take to prevent or at least delay the onset of an outbreak that could escalate beyond control without everyone's involvement. The use of scapegoats during a crisis is less likely to occur; response authorities can devote more of their attention to managing the disaster rather than managing their image; and members of the media may perform their public service mission of providing meaningful messages about personal safety, prevention of further dangerous exposure, and communicating public actions with advice from response agencies and disaster management experts.

Dr. Xue Lan, executive associate dean and professor at the School of Public Policy and Management, Tsinghua University, summarized China's challenges of facing a major public health crisis in the context of socioeconomic transition as a developing country and the criticality of focusing on prevention and preparedness as opposed to a reactive approach to crisis management. He identifies the critical elements—risk identification and assessment, risk communication to the public and decisionmakers, and risk mitigation and management—along with the structural reform requirements necessary to move from a reactive to a preventive crisis management system.[18]

Yet it is important to note that, whether developing or developed, large or small, "governments that fail to prepare for such disasters are preparing to fail."[19] The hurricanes on the Gulf Coast of the United States in 2005 demonstrate this point fully and have renewed awareness of the importance of deliberative preparedness planning at all levels of government and the private sector. Inadequate plans, failure to execute existing plans, lack of communication between sectors of the government, and poor response to misinformation caused a major disaster to

> *...whether developing or developed, large or small, "governments that fail to prepare for [such] disasters are preparing to fail."*

deteriorate into a crisis. Recovery from the accompanying crisis of confidence required

---

[17] Second- and third-level consequences are defined in Donald F. Thompson, "Terrorism and Domestic Response: Can DOD Help Get It Right? *Joint Force Quarterly* 40 , 1st Quarter, 2006, 18. Available at: <http://www.ndu.edu/inss/Press/jfq_pages/editions/i40/i40_forum_03.pdf>.

[18] Xue Lan, "Crisis Management in China: the Challenge of Transition," September 21, 2005, presentation for 2005 General Conference of the International Risk Governance Council. Available at: <http://www.irgc.org/_pdfs/WebsiteXUE.pdf>, accessed January 22, 2006.

[19] Jeb Bush, testimony before the House of Representatives Committee on Homeland Security, "Federalism and Disaster Response: Examining the Roles and Responsibilities of Local, State, and Federal Agencies," October 19, 2005, 4. Available at: <http://homeland.house.gov/files/TestimonyBush.pdf>.

the expenditure of resources at a level far exceeding what would have been required had adequate plans that could be efficiently executed been in place. An adequate response requires careful planning and training, and is essential to reassure the public and quickly restore some degree of normality after a disaster occurs.

Crisis Phases

Effective crisis management involves both *response phases* and *prevention phases*. The response phases have the goal of mitigating the effects of the incident, and include managing the emergency, limiting further damage, and recovering, or restoring well being. Prevention phases are broader and consist of actions that are taken both before a crisis develops and during all response phases. These actions include preparation, risk communication with the public, and learning.

Response Phases

The first response phase of managing any type of emergency is *detection*. It includes identifying opportunities for early warning of developing threats that can discriminate between normal background variability and a potential cluster of cases, identifying or developing a reporting mechanism of essential data elements, determining thresholds for actively collecting additional information, and utilizing opportunities to automate surveillance and early warning systems as much as is technologically feasible. An example of the detection phase for contagious diseases in mankind could be an automated disease data reporting system that identifies a number of cases of an infectious disease that exceeds the norm for a particular geographic area and automatically notifies a responsible party to begin an outbreak investigation. As the risk assessment and mitigation strategy tool advanced in this paper will show, detection, followed by an outbreak investigation, can lead to further assessment and identification of additional measures authorities might apply to reduce risk in a particular area even more. Risk reduction is a dynamic and iterative process that requires an appropriate framework if the positive impact on human and animal life is to be discernible.

The second and perhaps most important response phase, *limiting further damage*, involves three components: prompt initial response, immediate gathering of information to determine the scope of the incident or emergency, and rapid notification of other agencies that may be involved in reducing further damage or spread caused by the incident. These steps require that all agencies, authorities, and governments understand the first few steps that must be taken by each in response to an emergency and that all be prepared to respond immediately, especially in the face of incomplete information about the incident. It is also necessary to have considered the methods by which a rapid assessment may be performed so time will be devoted to collecting only the most essential data. Finally, this phase calls for immediate notifications to be made so that other agencies may prepare to respond if their assistance or resources are needed. The complex and challenging response phase requires that these tasks be performed simultaneously, since time is of the essence in the event of a communicable disease or a catastrophic event.

Interestingly, simultaneous performance of these steps is the opposite of the sequential method that is ingrained in scientists and in most executive managers and leaders. The tendency is to first collect all possible information that may shed light on the problem; then take initial response steps to correct the problem. After enough time has passed to detect improvement, a reassessment is performed to verify improvement, and adjustments to the response are made. Only when improvement is detected is notification made to higher authorities, peers, or the general public. The inadequacy of this process is obvious in a crisis setting, but the senior authorities who must make crisis management choices in an information vacuum are often in great need of practical experience in their decision making process.

In a small, contained emergency, this phase may be accomplished successfully if procedures and protocols for rapid assessment and notification have been developed, but most complex emergencies require that several people be devoted to rapid incident characterization and communicating needs and findings to other response agencies. Experienced crisis decisionmakers who can act effectively, given the lack of essential information, remain a rare commodity.

The third response phase is *recovery* from the disaster by restoring well being, which includes providing all resources necessary to meet emergency needs for food, water, medical care, housing, and restoring damaged infrastructure. This often requires extensive consideration of surge capacity—how to obtain additional supplies and equipment and hospital bed space to replace whatever was damaged in a natural disaster, locate additional healthcare workers to manage the additional injured or diseased persons, and find alternative delivery mechanisms of food, water, and equipment if the usual transportation infrastructure is damaged. In a large-scale disaster, many additional experts in public safety, engineering, transportation, communication, and mass care may be needed, as well as specialized equipment, supplies, and food.

Prevention Phases

Prevention phases are ongoing and transcend the pre-crisis and crisis phases. The most important step, *preparation*, includes developing comprehensive plans for prevention and response, ensuring crisis communication and information-sharing, identifying requirements for particular crises and the resources and capabilities to meet them, acknowledging capability gaps, and finding alternative sources for the personnel and equipment needed to provide such surge capacity.[20]

Another important prevention step is *risk communication* with the public, both before and during a crisis. Such communication often takes place through broadcast and print media,

---

[20] For a description of requirements-based deliberative planning in the medical sector, see Donald F. Thompson, "Terrorism and Domestic Response: Can DOD Help Get It Right? *Joint Force Quarterly,* 40, 1st Quarter, 2006, 18. Available at:
<http://www.ndu.edu/inss/Press/jfq_pages/editions/i40/i40_forum_03.pdf>.

and includes steps that people should take to protect themselves from danger. Authorities must accurately describe response steps that are being taken, the particular goals they desire to achieve with these steps, and the progress or lack thereof in achieving these goals. Information about steps the public should take to protect themselves must be provided in language that can be easily understood. A crucial component of this risk communication is that authorities must communicate that their response actions are based on what they currently know and that actions and recommendations may change as more information is learned. They must schedule multiple informational briefings or news conferences to indicate openness and transparency and to maintain trust.

An important facet of risk communication is that it is a key determinant of the degree of trust the public places in governmental authorities. It necessarily goes both ways, in that government authorities provide information to the public regarding what is known and unknown about the emergency. Likewise, response authorities must take in and address information from the public. This process is much more complex, since information from the public is often filtered through the media where the desire for market share often leads to sensationalism. Authorities must maintain awareness of the content of media broadcasts, and be prepared to provide accurate reports that confirm, clarify, or rebut that which is reported in the media.

Failure to address misinformation or to provide missing information quickly leads to questions about the transparency and competence of responsible authorities, and can prompt a crisis of confidence even in the context of a minor incident. If risk communication is effective, trust is built between the government and the governed. If it is ineffective or absent, then trust is lost and people may ignore important safety messages, or even do the opposite of what government authorities recommend. A positive example of such crisis communications can be found in the actions of New York City Mayor Rudolph Giuliani following the terrorist attacks against the World Trade Center on September 11, 2001. Negative examples abound, most recently in the response to Hurricane Katrina.

The third step of prevention is *learning*, where lessons are gleaned from a variety of experiences and applied to improve the effectiveness of future crisis management actions. This step includes both initial and ongoing training of response personnel so they will be as prepared as possible for their responsibilities in a crisis, and developing exercises that realistically test emergency plans and procedures. Appropriate government or industry officials should evaluate performance in these exercises and in actual crises according to accepted standards, so opportunities to improve response effectiveness can be identified at every occasion.

This learning process begins with thorough initial training of public and private sector individuals in their day-to-day responsibilities. In many jurisdictions, workers receive this training before they start to work so they have the skills they need to do their jobs, but in other locations, they are expected to learn these skills while on the job. A crucial breakdown in training and education occurs because these workers often are not trained in how their roles may change during an emergency response, what these new roles entail, action thresholds that clearly define the transition point from routine mode to emergency mode, the different communication and authority structures that often exist during an emergency response, the additional steps that must be taken to protect themselves during an emergency, and how to recognize when the emergency is over. Such training and education should include risk communication about any dangers to which they or their families might be exposed, any long-term physical and mental health effects to watch for, and where they should go to seek more information or help if they have particular concerns about potentially adverse physical or mental health conditions.[21]

A crucial aspect of pre-incident training is testing response preparedness in exercises that accurately replicate the pressures of accelerated timelines and missing information of a true emergency. Each emergency responder should be tested in several key areas: recognition of the emergency; initial notification of key response personnel or sounding the appropriate alarm; taking the first few emergency response steps; and rapid assessment of the scope of the emergency from their particular perspective and responsibilities. In other words, participants should not wait to be told what to do. Goals should be set for the timeliness of an acceptable response and the key elements of response that indicate satisfactory preparedness.

Once participants have demonstrated the ability to take the first few steps in a response, the emergency scenario should be complicated by the added requirement of coordinating the response with other sectors of business, industry, and government. For example, if the initial focus is a local public health agency, a more complex exercise might require coordination with law enforcement agencies, fire departments, environmental protection organizations, private industry (such as a major commercial air carrier), and the news media. Such a scenario requires interaction with persons from different institutional cultures who have different priorities, communicating and reporting styles, and measures of success. Their legal and regulatory requirements may be different, as may their acceptance of uncertainty. Lack of experience and comfort in working with persons from other response sectors during a major incident is a cause of the inefficient, ineffective emergency responses that are often observed. Communication barriers, coordination obstacles, and unsuspected flaws in complex response plans can be identified and proactively addressed during planned communications and tabletop exercises, so they do not first become apparent in an actual emergency, leading to unnecessary loss of life, loss of confidence of the public, and loss of stability of the government.

These prevention and response phases are critical elements of effective crisis management and prevention. Without adequate prevention efforts, a communicable disease outbreak can rapidly spread and develop into an epidemic. Without a suitable response plan, an epidemic is more likely to become a pandemic. Response and

---

[21] In the United States, an example of emergency response communication and authority structure is the Incident Command System used by the Federal Emergency Management Agency (FEMA) as part of the National Incident Management System. For further details, see <http://www.dhs.gov/dhspublic/interapp/press_release/press_release_0363.xml>.

prevention planning is relatively inexpensive when compared to the social, political, and economic disruption that results from losing control over a disease process with the risk magnitude of an influenza pandemic. Most importantly, prevention and response phases are aimed at the most important element of cooperative crisis management: preventing loss of life.

Section Three
Factors Affecting Prevention Strategies

Effective crisis management requires an understanding of the vulnerabilities one encounters in a particular geographic and political setting. Prevention and response efforts must be carefully focused and prioritized, so that limited resources can be applied efficiently. This requires that risks be assessed, vulnerable points identified, and actions taken that are most likely to mitigate these risks. A few of these actions may eliminate risk completely, but in most cases risk management techniques are applied where each effort provides some small degree of risk reduction. As similar efforts are applied across infrastructure, response, and transparency domains, noticeable risk reduction can be accomplished.[22]

Risk factors for communicable disease transmission are many and varied.[23] Some are immutable, such as geographic, environmental, and climatic features, while others are manmade and can be influenced (although with difficulty), such as population density, agricultural and industrial practices, and population movement characteristics. Understanding the contribution of these factors to local disease transmission risk not only allows actions to be taken that will reduce that risk but also improves international transparency as all users become familiar with the steps necessary for risk reduction.

Risk factors for spread of a communicable disease focus on the interaction and movement patterns of animal reservoirs, susceptible persons and infected persons. *Animal reservoirs* are those animals that may carry a particular bacterial or viral infection without showing signs of illness, or that may die of the infection. Rats carry the bacterium *Yersinia pestis*, the cause of bubonic plague, and ducks carry the avian influenza virus A/H5N1, but neither appears to suffer from the infections. Other animal reservoirs, however, infected with these same pathogens, may become sick and die from the disease, and may transmit the infection to other animals or to humans before they die. Examples include rabbits that are infected with *Francisella tularensis*, the bacterial cause of tularemia, and chickens

---

[22] Raymond Decker, "Homeland Security: A Risk Management Approach Can Guide Preparedness Efforts," GAO 02-208T (Washington, DC: Government Accountability Office, October 31, 2001).

[23] Multiple sources, including 58th World Health Assembly, "Revision of the International Health Regulations," May 23, 2005, World Health Organization, 45–48. Available at: <http://www.who.int/gb/ebwha/pdf_files/WHA58/WHA58_3-en.pdf>; World Health Organization, "Global Influenza Preparedness Plan," 2005. Available at: <http://www.who.int/csr/resources/publications/influenza/WHO_CDS_CSR_GIP_2005_5/en/>; World Health Organization, "Responding to the Avian Influenza Pandemic Threat: Recommended Strategic Actions," 2005. Available at: <http://www.who.int/csr/resources/publications/influenza/WHO_CDS_CSR_GIP_2005_8/en/index htm>; Food and Agriculture Organization, World Organization for Animal Health, "A Global Strategy for the Progressive Control of Highly Pathogenic Avian Influenza (HPAI)," May 2005. Available at: <http://www.fao.org/ag/againfo/resources/documents/empres/AI_globalstrategy.pdf>; U.S. Department of Health and Human Services, "HHS Pandemic Influenza Plan," November 2005. Available at: <http://www.hhs.gov/pandemicflu/plan/>; The White House, "National Strategy for Pandemic Influenza," November 2005. Available at: <http://www.whitehouse.gov/homeland/pandemic-influenza html>.

that become infected with avian influenza virus A/H5N1 from wild waterfowl and transmit the virus to other domestic chickens or to humans with whom they come into close contact. Many bacterial, viral, and parasitic infections are transmitted to humans by arthropod vectors, usually by blood-feeding ticks and insects, but a discussion of the epidemiology and transmission dynamics of these diseases is beyond the scope of this paper.[24]

Disease transmission risk factors include movement of both humans and animal reservoirs, since a pathogen may infect an animal or person in one location and then be transmitted to a distant location by air, ground, or water. Another important communicable disease risk factor is occupational exposure, as in the case of avian influenza, where poultry workers and persons who keep small domestic flocks of chickens are at higher risk for exposure from an animal source, and in SARS where healthcare workers at high risk for acquiring respiratory and blood-borne infections in the healthcare setting tragically were infected with the virus in 2003 and transmitted it to others.[25]

Due to the forces of globalization and easy international movement, risk factors in one country must be considered by countries on the other side of the earth. Rapid advances in international air travel allow persons incubating diseases to move around the globe before they even realize that they are sick, putting countries at risk that may be a great distance from the original source of the disease. Growth in international commerce and an increasingly internationalized food supply, coupled with a decrease in trade restrictions between neighboring countries, make it easier for microbes, disease-causing insects, and infected animals to travel around the world in as short a time as 24 hours. Action or inaction on an infectious disease outbreak in its country of origin now has global consequences.

> *Due to the forces of globalization and easy international movement, risk factors in one country must be considered by countries on the other side of the earth.*

Risk Factors

There are five general categories of risk factors that must be considered, evaluated, and addressed to either prevent or mitigate the spread of a contagious disease. These categories include: (1) ecological, (2) infrastructure, (3) response, (4) transparency, and (5) disease-specific outbreak and transmission factors. These factors lay the foundation for a risk assessment methodology and strategy for mitigation. In the prevention phase discussed previously, ecological and infrastructure factors are most salient. In the response phase of a crisis, response and disease outbreak transmission factors become

---

[24] Those interested in further information may start, for example, with José Ribeiro and Jesus Valenzuela, "Vector Biology," in *Tropical Infectious Diseases: Principles, Pathogens, and Practice*, Richard Guerrant et al., eds. (Philadelphia: Elsevier, 2005).

[25] Timothy Brooks, *Behind the Mask: How the World Survived SARS* (Washington, DC: American Public Health Association, 2005), 76–77.

more prominent. Transparency factors transcend both the prevention and response phases and are weighted accordingly. Appendix A provides the list of risk assessment and mitigation factors with a weighting scale (risk score) that can be used when conducting the self-assessment. Minimum and maximum scores are provided for each category and become useful when evaluating results and determining priorities for intervention. The relative value of these scores in terms of actual risk will be discussed in Section 4.

Ecological Factors

Ecological factors are those concerning population density, population composition and climatic features that favor disease transmission and are generally immutable. For example, a population density factor may be the degree of human interaction within a population group. Person-to-person transmission of a disease increases when humans are in close proximity. Urban, suburban, or rural environments contribute to the risk for disease transmission based on human interaction. It is important to note that no single factor will determine an at-risk population. Therefore, a rural population with minimal hygiene practices may be at higher risk for disease transmission than a suburban population with sound hygiene practices. Despite these better practices, the suburban population may be likely to transmit the disease to larger numbers of people, due to the increased opportunity for contact between an infected person and a susceptible person. Both populations may require intervention, though specific intervention measures may vary.

Another ecological factor concerns the population composition of the environment. Immunosuppressed populations may be at higher risk for communicable respiratory diseases. Children, pregnant women, persons with HIV/AIDS, the elderly, and those who are severely malnourished are more susceptible to disease and would likely experience an increased death rate. However, overall risk scores might be reduced if these populations had been predetermined to be at elevated risk, surveillance for diseases was enhanced, and early access to healthcare services was provided.

Climate is yet another ecological factor that affects disease transmission. The temperature and humidity of tropical climates are more favorable to transmission of many more bacterial and parasitic diseases than in arid or temperate climates. Speculation exists that the burden of tropical diseases and parasitic infestations that flourish in moist and warm climates were a barrier to widespread population growth in the tropics, and led to settlement in temperate zones in Eurasia.[26] An exception to this tropical disease transmission factor is seasonal influenza, since its transmission actually increases in a cool, dry climate.

Infrastructure Factors

Infrastructure factors cover the spectrum of basic animal husbandry practices, public health disease surveillance systems, and healthcare delivery capacity. Generally, these

---

[26] William McNeill, *Plagues and People* (New York: Doubleday, 1976), 74.

include the presence of animal-human interaction, effective human disease surveillance processes, access to remote populations who may be infected, and the need for external assistance to detect, investigate, respond to, and control a disease outbreak or prevent new cases. The ability to rapidly make and verify a disease diagnosis is an important infrastructure factor, since it is essential for clinical management to be more effective and identify the most appropriate steps that must be quickly taken to interrupt transmission.

The ability of an effective healthcare delivery system to safely manage highly infectious pathogens is also a critical factor in disease prevention and mitigation. If a hospital has no reverse-isolation infection control patient rooms or there is poor healthcare worker compliance with infection control principles, hospital transmission of infectious diseases is much more likely to occur.

Effective public risk communication and interagency coordination are equally important risk factors. Effective risk communication between government agencies and the public is necessary to provide reassurance and instructions on personal steps that should be taken to protect from a disease. Likewise, effective preparedness and response planning requires successful communication and interagency coordination between all local and central government agencies, including agriculture, veterinary medicine, public health, education, transportation, commerce, communication, and security apparatuses. The enormous gap in communication and coordination between public health agencies and veterinary services in many countries is surprising, since animal-to-human transmission is the tipping point and lethal step toward person-to-person transmission of infectious diseases.

Response Factors

Response factors are those characteristics of agricultural and public health systems that are most highly correlated with successful management of disease outbreaks. Such characteristics rarely develop spontaneously in government agencies that do not have an emergency response role. With adequate attention, however, appropriate procedures can be put in place during the prevention stage of planning and can then be practiced so that an effective response to a disease outbreak quickly occurs. Some response factors are associated with the immediate actions that authorities must take, while others consist of data collection systems and procedures about disease surveillance and reporting. The critical success feature of an effective response, though, is coordination across every aspect and phase of response.

Rapid decisions must be made in the absence of crucial information, and response actions must be redirected and improved as that information becomes available. In the case of avian influenza, for example, local health authorities must identify animal reservoirs, disease transmission factors, and high-risk groups before an emergency occurs. Then, when the highly pathogenic virus is detected in migratory waterfowl, authorities can require that steps be taken to protect domestic poultry from coming into contact with migratory waterfowl, and human contact with domestic poultry can be minimized by appropriate biosecurity steps or eliminated altogether. Active case finding can be implemented to detect additional cases in wild and domestic bird populations, and active human respiratory disease surveillance can be initiated. If these steps are not taken, the risk of disease transmission greatly increases as response authorities waste precious time trying to figure out how to respond.

Other important response factors are associated with disease surveillance systems. These provide essential background and real-time disease data, so the first few cases of a disease may be rapidly detected and control efforts may be initiated. Included are surveillance systems for animal reservoirs, for presence of human disease, and for detecting disease cases in high-risk areas. Disease surveillance systems should be able to distinguish between mild and severe cases of a disease to allow for the more efficient prioritization of limited resources. Animal disease surveillance is particularly important. As part of a robust animal husbandry infrastructure, animal disease surveillance systems identify animal reservoirs for various diseases. This enables response authorities to take steps to protect domestic animal populations from wild populations as well as cull infected animal populations to minimize the spread of animal disease and reduce the risk of human exposure. The financial implications of such practices may be significant when such a program is first established, but the broad economic benefits of improved animal husbandry will often balance these costs in the long term.

In contrast to infrastructure factors, public communication and effective interagency response coordination depend on procedures and processes rather than on concrete physical items for assessment, and it is reasonable to assume that they can be more easily altered than can healthcare infrastructure or animal husbandry practices. If there is little evidence of coordinated crisis responses between officials at different levels of government and between government agencies, or if interagency cooperation occurs only during a crisis in response to pressure from senior government leaders or criticism from the media or other sources, a systemic weakness in crisis response is often present. An effective response requires rapid, coordinated action by all involved local and central government agencies with little confusion about roles and responsibilities, so time and effort are not wasted.

Transparency

Quick information-sharing is the hallmark of a successful response. All parties must understand their own roles and responsibilities and those of other parties. Each must know the likely steps that will be taken as an emergency incident response unfolds, and when information is identified that may improve or redirect steps being taken by other agencies, processes must be in place that allow this new information to quickly flow to those who need it. Because infectious diseases do not recognize borders, not only is information-sharing critical within a country, it is also crucial between states and within multilateral organizations that support their members at the international level.

Cooperative crisis management depends on such transparency. It is essential that the actions taken during a response and the effectiveness of these actions be apparent externally. Many nations will notice when another responsible member of the global community experiences an emergency and often will offer help—through direct technical assistance in responding to the emergency, if required, or perhaps through international finance or trade adjustments. Likewise, if the threat is an infectious disease, other countries, especially neighboring ones, will be attentive to the findings within the affected country and the actions being taken to bring it under control, enabling their leaders to take appropriate steps to protect their citizens and national security interests.

How countries react depends in large part on their confidence in the affected country's own assessment of the disease transmission risk and in how openly it shares information within and outside its own borders. Governance is a complicating factor: where poor living conditions,

> **How countries react depends in large part on their confidence in the affected country's own assessment of the disease transmission risk and in how openly it shares information within and outside its own borders.**

inadequately functioning societal infrastructure, inability to maintain law and order, and failure to respond to complex emergencies exist, [27] outside countries are likely to view an affected country's self-assessment with wariness and may take more drastic measures to protect their own citizens, which may or may not be warranted by the actual circumstances.

Seven factors can assist in determining confidence in another country's disease transmission risk assessment: (1) effective disease surveillance, (2) transparency in surveillance and its findings, (3) effective containment of disease outbreaks, (4) maintenance of public infrastructure, (5) maintenance of public trust, (6) ability of the media to report on these factors, and (7) timely, accurate reporting to the WHO and other multilateral organizations.

- **Disease surveillance.** Effective surveillance will accurately identify animal and human diseases of concern, or syndromes that may suggest the presence of these diseases as early as possible and will include processes to promptly report findings to responsible authorities for collection, reporting, and action. This requires knowledge of the background occurrence of diseases according to seasonal and geographic patterns.

- **Transparency in surveillance.** Surveillance reporting must be timely, accurate, and open. Local authorities should openly communicate both positive news and causes for concern to their superiors for information and for appropriate action. Portions of these reports should be open to the media, within the scope of reasonable parameters that protect the identity of individuals and do not impair response. Local and national authorities should provide regular updates, especially during an emergency. If this communication occurs only when local or international pressure is exerted, it suggests that government officials recognize neither the benefits of such information-sharing nor the unintended consequences

---

[27] Donald MacMillan, "Model Describing the Effect of Employment of the United States Military in a Complex Emergency," *Prehospital and Disaster Medicine*, September/October 2005, 282–289.

of such reticence upon national economies via decreased tourism, declining foreign direct investment, and instability of capital markets.

- **Effective containment.** When steps are taken to rapidly identify additional cases and those who may have been exposed, this suggests that proper governance is in place and substantive public health planning has occurred. Further positive indicators of effective containment include appropriate isolation techniques in hospitals that effectively protect patients, healthcare workers, and the general public from disease transmission in these high-risk settings.

- **Maintenance of public infrastructure.** A crucial indicator of quality organization is an orderly society that effectively recovers from stresses to the system caused by natural disasters and other emergencies. This includes the protection and maintenance of critical infrastructure necessary to provide for public safety, such as police, fire protection, emergency medical services, hospitals, water, electricity, and natural gas. Food must continue to be available in local markets, and electricity and telephone service should be quickly restored in an emergency. Even such a seemingly inconsequential activity such as garbage collection in urban settings must be included.

- **Public trust.** National and local governments depend on public trust to maintain their authority. When there is confidence in government, the governed will tend to comply with instructions on self-protection steps. Without such confidence, they will often either actively or passively protest, such as fleeing when directed to submit to quarantine as occurred in Hong Kong in response to SARS control efforts.[28]

- **Ability of media to report.** An open media is an essential partner in an effective, responsive government, even though criticism of government officials appears to be detrimental at times. While media outlets may occasionally irresponsibly generate misinformation, the adjustments that leaders make to improve governance, accuracy, and openness often compensate for perceived loss of credibility.

- **Good reporting to the WHO, FAO, and OIE.** Authorities should report accurately to the WHO, FAO, and OIE, since such additional information increases not only the effectiveness of these multinational organizations, but also the respect of governmental authorities in the international arena. WHO and other agencies should be permitted to visit outbreak locations in order to assist, verify, and validate findings and containment actions being taken.

---

[28] Stephen Ng, "The Mystery of Amoy Gardens," in Loh and Civic Exchange, eds., 97.

This category of risk factors is tailored specifically to the particular disease process that is threatening the population. It deals with whether or not the disease is present in a geographic area and with pathogen characteristics in the actual environment in which the risk assessment is being performed. Some use the term *hot zone* to describe the geographic location of an initial disease outbreak. This definition may apply to a few kilometers around a particular site if the area can be well demarcated, or it may be broadly applied to an entire nation, region, or continent. It is clear that until the risk for transmission of the infection is minimized by actions that contain the spread of the pathogen, this hot zone area will be large. As disease transmission is brought under control, the size of the hot zone will shrink. The *warm zone* will be that geographic area in immediate proximity to the hot zone, and its size will reflect the ease with which people or infected animals can move into or out of the hot zone. Transmission barriers such as relatively impassable terrain provide some degree of safety, though these have largely been overcome by international air travel. The *cold zone* will be all other areas of the world.

Countries in and near outbreaks of infectious diseases may perform a risk assessment using the factors described in this section and may thereby identify mutable risk factors that may be conducive to mitigation steps. In Section 5 we demonstrate the utility of this methodology using avian influenza as it manifests itself today in a case study.

Some pathogen characteristics in a geographic location change over time, in that the virulence of an organism may change where the severity of illness caused by a bacterium or a virus may either increase or decrease.[29] Other characteristics may vary as well, such as the ease with which the organism is transmitted between animal reservoirs, between the reservoir and humans, or from person to person. The unique characteristics of the pathogen in its reservoir, the behaviors of the reservoir, and the ease with which the disease is transmitted from person to person have a profound impact on the steps that must be taken to effectively interrupt transmission, so a realistic risk assessment must consider these factors for each particular disease. The example used to demonstrate the methodology in this paper is highly pathogenic avian influenza A/H5N1 as known in late 2005. The methodology applies to almost any other human respiratory pathogen that can be transmitted from person to person such as tuberculosis, *Mycoplasma* pneumonia, smallpox, pneumonic plague, and many others, though the opportunities for intervention may be different.

Effective interruption of disease transmission requires that steps be taken at multiple points so that an outbreak may quickly be brought under control.[30] Transmission between reservoir animals should be reduced to minimize the presence of the pathogen in the

---

[29] *Virulence* is the quality of being poisonous, or the power of evoking disease in a given host.

[30] World Health Organization, "Pandemic Influenza Draft Protocol for Rapid Response and Containment," 27 January 2006, 12-13. Available at: <http://www.who.int/csr/disease/avian_influenza/guidelines/RapidResponse.pdf>.

environment, contact between reservoir animals and humans should be minimized or eliminated completely, and exposed humans should be carefully monitored for signs of disease. Those incubating an infection should be kept from contact with unexposed persons and should be treated as rapidly as possible, both to reduce the severity of the developing disease and to reduce the likelihood that it will be transmitted to others. A disease with a long incubation period is more difficult to control, since persons incubating the infection continue to move about and may expose many others to the infection before they become so ill that they alter their activities and stay home.[31]

A disease that is continuously present in an area often has successfully adapted to the local environmental and biological conditions and therefore is much more difficult to eradicate or control than one that has been recently introduced. On the other hand, a newly identified pathogen may be more difficult to control, since its animal reservoir, if any, may be unknown, the mechanism of transmission to humans may be poorly understood, and the frequency and ease of person-to-person transmission is often not clear until medical personnel and scientists become familiar with its clinical characteristics. The resulting disease may be difficult to diagnose, and it may require unusual medications or supportive care to prevent severe illness and death. Each of these unknowns raises the risk of person-to-person transmission, requires more intensive study and action to understand, and reduces the likelihood of quickly bringing an outbreak under control.

Several specific pathogen characteristics warrant further discussion in regard to the degree of disease transmission risk they pose. A pathogen that quickly causes severe illness and death in its animal reservoir is at a lower risk for transmission than one that causes a mild illness or no illness at all. For example, highly pathogenic avian influenza A/H5N1 quickly causes death in its goose and chicken reservoirs, and so its presence is more apparent in these populations since such large die-offs of birds are noticed by people in the vicinity. Conversely, the same pathogen causes little or no detectable illness in some populations of ducks, so it can be spread by such ducks, whose infected excreta causes widespread contamination of the environment, leading to infection of other migratory waterfowl species. In other populations of ducks, the pathogen is highly pathogenic and just as fatal as in many geese and chicken. This complex pattern of survival in different animal reservoirs, and the potential for global spread via migratory waterfowl or by smuggling or legitimate trade of infected birds, suggests that this particular virus may be impossible to eradicate, and efforts to reduce transmission in mankind must be directed elsewhere.

The opposite risk exists for a disease pathogen that quickly causes severe illness and death in mankind. A pathogen that is efficiently transmitted from person to person and causes severe illness will quickly overwhelm the healthcare delivery system, causing profound disruption to society and leading to dramatic efforts by individuals to protect themselves from infection. Fear and panic historically have caused massive population

---

[31] The incubation period is the time between initial exposure to the pathogen and the time when symptoms of the disease develop.

movements as people flee areas that they think are more dangerous. Societal infrastructure is put at risk, shortages in basic services such as food and water may develop, and authorities may have difficulty maintaining law and order. Disease transmission may actually increase in the face of such disorder due to crowding and decreased availability of clean water and adequate sanitation. A pathogen that slowly causes a mild disease to develop is often easier to control, since public health officials have more time to identify exposed contacts and educate the public about protective steps that reduce the risk of infection.

A pathogen that leads to a disease with similar characteristics to other diseases in the environment is often more difficult to control, since recognition of its presence in the environment may be delayed. A novel illness may be unapparent if the usual rate of illnesses with similar signs and symptoms is high in a particular region.

Characteristics of persons at greatest risk of exposure vary with each pathogen, and have a significant impact on efforts to interrupt transmission and control an outbreak. Surveillance and control of these groups is crucial, since they may put many others at risk for disease transmission. For example, commercial and domestic agricultural workers, who are at an increased risk for exposure to avian influenza, may travel from rural farms to urban markets while incubating disease. Healthcare workers are also at particular risk for any respiratory or blood-borne pathogen, and usually take precautions for personal protection. Precautions may break down, however, due to inattention, as occurred with SARS patients at the Prince of Wales hospital in Hong Kong.[32] Hospital workers who care for patients with communicable diseases may unwittingly transmit pathogens from an infected patient to other patients whose immune systems are incapable of fighting off an infection, and to their family members and other contacts outside of the hospital.

Cases of the disease that develop in persons with unclear travel histories are particularly difficult to trace to their origin, raising the risk for further person-to-person transmission. International travel increases the number of opportunities for exposing others, the number of pathogens to which an ill person may have been exposed, and the likelihood that the illness will be misdiagnosed by a healthcare clinician who is not familiar with all the diseases in a distant country or region of exposure.

The five major risk factors just described constitute the basis for the risk assessment tool that will be described in Section 4. Such a tool will permit local and national authorities to evaluate their particular environment and determine, as well as prioritize, where scarce resources should be applied to mitigate risk. But first, a few words about information-sharing are in order.

Information-sharing

Because disease threats have global consequences, unprecedented cooperation and information-sharing are needed to maintain the free flow of people and goods, while

---

[32]Brooks, *Behind the Mask: How the World Survived SARS,* 53.

simultaneously reassuring both governments and the public that they are safe. Every country desires to provide opportunities for its citizens and to encourage economic growth, while avoiding the risks of instability or lawlessness that threatens its vital interests. Economic growth often requires open borders so people and goods may move freely, while security and stability require early detection of threats and prompt protective action. Animal and human disease threats are particularly difficult to identify, since they are often present at a background level throughout the world, varying according to geography and season.

Most human health security threats are recognized by the WHO in the International Health Regulations, and include cholera, plague, and yellow fever. Other infectious diseases have assumed the same or greater level of importance, due to their transmissibility and lethality, including SARS, viral hemorrhagic fevers such as Ebola and Marburg, and avian influenza. A major criterion for concern is the threat from an emerging infectious disease that is unusual, unexpected, or from an unknown cause. When the method of transmission and the incubation period are unknown, such as was the case with SARS when it was first discovered in early 2003, control measures are difficult and public health authorities often overreact to protect the population. WHO guidelines highlight a number of factors that must be considered both domestically and internationally to help to determine the threat from an infectious disease.[33]

Animal disease surveillance findings are coordinated internationally by the FAO and the OIE. These organizations do not coordinate these animal disease findings with the human disease findings from the WHO, a serious omission that can lead to significant delays in disease recognition and response. A call has gone out to bring these global health management players

> **These organizations [FAO and OIE] do not coordinate...animal disease findings with the human disease findings from the WHO, a serious omission that can lead to significant delays in disease recognition and response.**

together in managing emerging infectious diseases, a need that is particularly important as avian influenza spreads around the globe.[34]

Countries need reporting systems and rules to identify these risks, collect these reports, and take appropriate actions to investigate and control further disease transmission. Finally, countries need mechanisms to share information about internal disease outbreaks and the effectiveness of control measures, since these factors will often drive behavior by other countries to protect themselves from perceived disease threats.

---

[33] 58th World Health Assembly, "Revision of the International Health Regulations."

[34] T. Kuiken, F.A. Leighton, R.A.M. Fouchier, J.W. LeDuc, J.S. M. Peiris, A. Schudel, K. Stöhr, and A.D. M. E. Osterhaus, "Pathogen Surveillance in Animals," *Science* 309 , September 9, 2005, 1680–1681.

Domestic Information Collection

Public health officials often rely on a combination of passive and active surveillance systems. Passive systems involve health centers, hospitals, and doctors, that are expected to notify local public health offices of certain disease cases when diagnosed in patients. Active surveillance involves public health staffs calling on doctors and hospitals to inquire if cases of interest have been seen. Both methods have drawbacks: the first is unreliable, since it requires doctors and hospitals to take the time to report cases, while the second is very time-consuming and slow. Data collection sometimes is improved during an outbreak, since media coverage reminds healthcare workers of the need to report cases and potential patients of their need to seek medical attention.

International Information Collection

Information about diseases that may be occurring at a distance is more difficult to obtain but is crucial in today's global economy. Disease reporting is often an internal issue, and reports of new disease outbreaks may take weeks to reach international partners. The reasons for slow reporting are many, including inadequate disease surveillance and reporting policies, inadequate surveillance and reporting technology, insufficient local and national emphasis on collection and reporting, as well as bureaucratic obstacles to sharing data. Countries must identify those diseases and conditions that justify the additional effort required to report since many diseases are common and do not pose a local, national, or international health security threat.

Risks of Sharing Information

Some countries may be reluctant to share such detailed information out of fear that it may cast them in a negative light in the international community, or lead to domestic confusion, instability, panic, and economic loss from decreased travel. The SARS experience is illustrative of the negative consequences of withholding facts, which belittles the ability of citizens to act rationally and undermines public trust in the government. Citizens typically trust the government to tell them the truth and to refrain from generating panic. Once officials have hidden facts even once, they may never again enjoy the full confidence of citizens. The lack of sharing information also leads to more disease spread, since other hospitals and public health officials may not have any warning about the presence of a highly contagious infection. Precautions against disease may be inadequate, causing the disease to spread.[35]

Risks of Withholding Information

Inadequate communication and cooperation from a government may lead to undesirable actions by its own citizens. Lack of transparency by the Hong Kong government early in the response to SARS caused the public to take the initiative. Many parents withdrew their children from school and administrators voluntarily closed schools, while the media

---

[35] Alexis Lau, "The Numbers Trail: What the Data Tells Us," in Loh and Civic Exchange, eds., 81–83.

led a fund-raising campaign to purchase adequate protective clothing for front-line hospital staff. Businesses launched informational campaigns to inform themselves and their overseas colleagues of the situation.[36] These events actually underlined the ineffectiveness of the government and its indifference to the public.

If information is withheld, other countries may find it necessary to act to protect their own population and interests from perceived risks that may originate in a country affected by an infectious disease outbreak. Such actions may or may not be warranted and could be partially or completely avoided if the affected country openly communicated, both domestically and internationally, information about local risks, intervention steps, and outcomes. Negative actions may include closing international borders, denying entry of travelers from the affected country, issuing advisories that discourage travel to the affected region, or even reducing trade with the affected country.

---

[36] Michael E. DeGolyer, "How the Stunning Outbreak of Disease Led to a Stunning Outbreak of Dissent," in Loh and Civic Exchange, eds., 124.

Section Four
Developing a Risk Assessment and Mitigation Strategy

Cooperative crisis management in the international context demands a common lexicon and methodology for evaluating risk, taking preventive action, and responding to an actual communicable disease outbreak. As governments consider necessary and reasonable steps to protect the welfare of their citizens and livelihoods from such an outbreak, they look to other countries to better understand the strategic international and regional environment. Several countries in one part of the world acting in ways that appear out of the ordinary or not taking actions that others deem appropriate may be cause for concern. Distant countries probably will be prompted by such inconsistencies to pay closer attention and to reassess their own priorities and vulnerabilities in the context of skepticism, concern, and uncertainty. This reassessment may involve formal diplomatic contact, unofficial communications with treaty, coalition, and trading partners, or simply observing open media reports. Data and information acquired (or not acquired) during this reassessment will often have a direct bearing on security actions each nation takes. These data may reassure decisionmakers, putting them more at ease, or it may cause alarm and lead to an escalation in protective actions. A common understanding of risk factors and response steps will greatly support international cooperative efforts to minimize the effects of crises, be they natural disasters, public health emergencies, or the consequences of a terrorist attack.

If one takes history as a mirror and looks to the future, the 1918–1919 influenza pandemic provides a stark perspective on a potential avian influenza pandemic. The SARS experience adds a more recent and humanly felt quality to international community concerns. The uncertainty regarding the likelihood of an avian influenza outbreak, coupled with the grave consequences if the virus became easily transmissible among humans, provides the backdrop for today's international focus on avian influenza and the tool provided here for developing a risk assessment and mitigation strategy.

The environmental, ecological, and infrastructure factors developed in the previous section apply equally well for SARS, plague, tularemia, viral hemorrhagic fevers, West Nile fever, and many other pathogens, though minor modification of these factors may be appropriate and the weighting criteria may vary somewhat. Disease outbreak, transmission, and response factors as described in the previous section and in Appendix A will broadly apply to any communicable disease and are often relevant to preparation for and response to natural disasters. The transparency factors are relevant to many settings where one group, nation, or organization may need to consider the actions of another.

Since communicable diseases are spread either person to person or via an insect or animal vector, geographic proximity to the initial disease location has always been vitally important for communicable disease transmission. In today's international business

37

environment, though, other factors may be just as important, since insect and animal vectors are mobile, and exposed persons often pass through an incubation period before the clinical symptoms of the disease may develop. During this incubation period, infected persons may travel great distances, putting others at risk and transmitting the disease far beyond its originating location.

The particular transmission risks of each of these factors may be quantified in scientific studies, but the practical application of such detail is limited, due to the variety of risk factors, social characteristics, and ecological variables. In contrast, a pragmatic, qualitative disease risk assessment process is useful from several perspectives. First, it allows agencies and authorities who may be responsible for protecting their population from infectious disease threats to identify features of their particular local environment that may increase transmission risks, take focused steps to prevent spread of an infectious disease, and apply efforts and resources in the most expeditious manner.

Second, it highlights vulnerabilities in that local environment that may call for immediate attention when an outbreak first occurs, so that the outbreak may quickly be brought under control. This reduces the amount of unnecessary time that elapses before active intervention. Third, an internationally accepted, standardized infectious disease risk assessment methodology allows agencies, authorities, and countries that may be geographically distant to determine the degree of disease transmission risk within the outbreak area and evaluate what, if any, steps are reasonable to take to prevent the disease from being transmitted into the location for which they are responsible. This final step is currently very difficult, since few objective criteria have been defined and accurate information is rarely available. The perceived risk is often very subjective and is often largely based on excessive speculation in the face of fear, misunderstanding and pressure to take action.

An internationally recognized, valid, objective risk assessment methodology provides both a self-assessment tool and a more accurate process for determining risk of international disease transmission. It supports local risk mitigation steps and reduces the likelihood that inappropriate steps will be taken on the international stage that may have negative economic or security impacts. Because a risk assessment and mitigation strategy is relational—that is, the outcome of actions taken or not taken in one country can have an impact (either positive or negative) in other countries—it is essential to place disease transmission risk zones in a geographical context.

Avian Influenza Pandemic Risk Factors and WHO Phases

The current concerns about HPAI A/H5N1 have prompted a careful reexamination of previous outbreaks, including the source and timing of the virus that caused each pandemic, the mechanisms of spread, the clinical symptoms caused by each virus, and the genetic characteristics of each virus. The likelihood exists of genetic modification due to antigenic drift, shift, or reassortment of the influenza RNA viral genome, since such modifications are regularly observed in nature.[37] The difficulty comes in predicting the actual present pandemic risk from these potential changes. If such genetic changes occur that increase the transmissibility between persons, this new virus subtype could quickly spread from person to person, causing a global pandemic. There is presently little scientific basis for predicting whether the current HPAI A/H5N1 virus will become pandemic, since none of the known pandemic influenza events of the past 87 years seem to have much in common with the current H5N1 situation. It is also difficult to predict if these viruses are even moving toward solving the fundamental challenge of switching and propagating in a different host.[38]

Previous influenza pandemics have been due to different influenza A virus subtypes. The 1918 pandemic virus was caused by an H1N1 subtype; the 1957 Asian virus pandemic was due to an H2N2 subtype; and the 1968 Hong Kong virus pandemic was due to an H3N2 subtype.[39] These latter two pandemic viruses were avian/human reassortants, where several avian gene segments reassorted with the human adapted virus that was then circulating. Recent research suggests, however, that the 1918 pandemic virus did not develop as a reassortant virus, but was instead an avian virus that adapted to humans.[40]

The range of mammals susceptible to influenza is great. Humans, chickens, ducks, quail, geese, felids, rodents, and swine are just some of the species susceptible to influenza A. The mechanisms of the spread of influenza virus between animals and humans are very complex, due to the virus' widespread presence in many animal hosts. The virus could be transferred within and between countries by reservoir animals, such as domestic ducks and chickens or migratory birds, by movement of humans, or by inanimate objects such as shoes and boots. Good biosecurity measures at poultry farms can reduce spread by movement of poultry or poultry products, and careful cleansing and disinfection of footwear can help protect from inadvertent farm cross-contamination. Live poultry markets are both a reservoir and an amplifier of infection and are suspected to play a role

---

[37] *Antigenic drift* is when small genetic changes occur in the influenza virus over time that produce new strains that are no longer recognized by the body's immune system. This allows reinfection to occur with the same viral subtype. Most people who have been exposed to circulating influenza viruses have partial immunity to a new strain that comes about by antigenic drift. *Antigenic shift* is when an abrupt, major change occurs in the influenza virus, leading to new hemagglutinin and/or neuraminidase proteins and a new viral subtype. Most people have little to no immune protection against such a new virus. Source: Centers for Disease Control and Prevention, "The Influenza (Flu) Viruses." Available at: < http://www.cdc.gov/flu/about/fluviruses htm>, accessed January 10, 2006. *Reassortment* of genetic material occurs when a host (bird, pig, or person) is infected with two or more different influenza virus subtypes at the same time. Segments of the RNA virus genome can be shared between these subtypes, leading to a new subtype (the reassortant). Source: Centers for Disease Control and Prevention, "Transmission of Avian Influenza Viruses Between Animals and People." Available at: <http://www.cdc.gov/flu/avian/gen-info/transmission.htm>, accessed January 10, 2006.

[38] Jeffery K. Taubenberger and David M. Morens, "Influenza Revisited," *Emerging Infectious Diseases* 12, no. 1, January 2006, 1–2.

[39] Edwin Kilbourne, "Influenza Pandemics of the 20th Century," *Emerging Infectious Diseases* 12, no. 1, January 2006, 9–14.

[40] Jeffery K. Taubenberger et al., "Characterization of the 1918 influenza virus polymerase genes," *Nature* 437, 2005, 889–893.

in the maintenance and spread of HPAI A/H5N1 virus in Asia.[41] Backyard flocks are common in Asia, yet are not subject to any biosecurity measures. Fighting cocks are often transported long distances, and may play a role in spreading the infection and in its transmission to humans.[42]

Despite the difficulty in identifying a viral subtype and strain that may cause any future pandemic, much of the preparatory work in recent years has been directed toward vaccine development. There is an unquestionable need to modernize vaccine development methodologies and to construct and upgrade production facilities so that vaccines may be quickly developed. Until a candidate pandemic vaccine strain has been identified, however, it is premature to expend large amounts of resources toward vaccine development. In a similar fashion, the use of antiviral medications is limited, since these drugs often shorten the clinical course of an infection by only one day. These challenges—a complex reservoir and transmission pattern, rapidly changing genetic characteristics, and limited availability of pharmaceutical interventions—imply that alternative methods of prevention and control must be developed.

The WHO has developed non-pharmaceutical interventions that serve to reduce exposure of susceptible persons to infectious agents, based on historical infection control practices used to control many agents. These interventions focus on:

- limiting international spread of the virus by travel screening and restrictions
- reducing spread within national and local populations by isolation and treatment of ill persons, monitoring and possible quarantine of exposed populations, and social distancing measures such as cancellation of mass gatherings and closure of schools
- reducing the individual's risk of infection by good hand hygiene and disinfection.[43,44]

Details about these specific measures may be found in the sources cited, while the current risk assessment and risk mitigation methodology outlined in this paper helps to identify some of the areas where such measures should be taken.

---

[41] Richard Fielding et al, "Avian Influenza Risk Perception," *Emerging Infectious Diseases* 11, no. 5, May 2005, 677–682.

[42] Robert Webster et al., "H5N1 Outbreaks and Enzootic Influenza," *Emerging Infectious Diseases* 12, no. 1, January 2006, 3–8.

[43] World Health Organization Writing Group, "Nonpharmaceutical Interventions for Pandemic Influenza, International Measures," *Emerging Infectious Diseases* 12, no. 1, January 2006, 81–87.

[44] Ibid., 88–94.

Summary of WHO Global Pandemic Phases[45]

New Phases	Overarching Public Health Goals
Interpandemic period	
Phase 1: No influenza virus subtypes have been detected in humans. An influenza virus that has caused human infection may be present in animals. If present in animals, the risk of human infection or disease is considered to be low.	Strengthen influenza pandemic preparedness at the global, regional, national and sub-national level.
Phase 2: No new influenza virus subtypes have been detected in humans. However, a circulating animal influenza virus subtype poses a substantial risk of human disease.	Minimize the risk of transmission to humans; detect and report such transmission rapidly if it occurs.
Pandemic alert period	
Phase 3: Human infections(s) with a new subtype, but no human-to-human spread, or at most rare instances of spread to a close contact.[a]	Ensure rapid characterization of the new virus subtype and early detection, notification and response to additional cases.
Phase 4: Small cluster(s) with limited human-to-human transmission but spread is highly localized, suggesting that the virus is not well adapted to humans.	Contain the new virus within limited foci or delay spread to gain time to implement preparedness measures, including vaccine development.
Phase 5: Larger cluster(s) but human-to-human spread still localized, suggesting that the virus is becoming increasingly better adapted to humans, but may not yet be fully transmissble (substantial pandemic risk)	Maximize efforts to contain or delay spread, to possibly avert a pandemic, and to gain time to implement pandemic response measure.
Pandemic period	
Phase 6: Pandemic: increased and substantial transmission in general public.[b]	Minimize the impact of the pandemic.

a The distinction between *phase 1* and *phase 2* is based on the risk of human infection or disease resulting from circulating strains in the animals The distinction is based on various factors and their relative importance according to current scientific knowledge Factors may include pathogenicity in animals and humans, occurrence in domesticated animals and livestock or only in wildlife, whether the virus is enzootic or epizootic, geographically localized or widespread, and/or other scientific parameters

b The distinction between *phase 3*, *phase 4* and *phase 5* is based on an assessment of the risk of a pandemic Various factors and their relative importance according to current scientific knowledge may be considered Factors may include rate of transmission, geographical location and spread, severity of illness, presence of genes from human strains (if derived from an animal strain), and/or other scientific parameters

The WHO has identified six pandemic phases and developed strategic actions linked to each prevention phase. The stated goals include:

- reducing opportunities for human infection
- strengthening the early warning system

[45] World Health Organization. "WHO global influenza preparedness plan: The role of WHO and recommendations for national measures before and during pandemics," WHO/CDS/CSR/GIP/2005.5 (Geneva: World Health Organization, 2005).

41

- containing or delaying spread at the source
- reducing morbidity, mortality, and social disruption.[46]

These phases focus on surveillance and response during the critical points where human transmissibility is possible and are reproduced here from the *WHO Global Influenza Preparedness Plan*. Our risk assessment methodology integrates these six WHO pandemic phases to provide a common reference point when prioritizing intervention strategy resources on a global level.

The WHO points out that the distinction between phase 1 and phase 2 is based on the risk of human infection or disease resulting from circulating animal strains of influenza virus, while the distinctions between phase 3, phase 4, and phase 5 are based on the assessment of the risk of a pandemic. This is the risk that is examined in the present study and risk assessment methodology, as becomes apparent in the avian influenza case study (Section 5).

A Risk Assessment and Mitigation Strategy Tool

The risk assessment and mitigation strategy tool we present in this paper permits local and national authorities, as well as international donor organizations and others, to evaluate a particular environment and determine where mitigation opportunities exist. In some geographic and political settings, for example, it may be possible to alter agricultural practices to reduce the risk that an infection may be transmitted from animals to man, while in other settings, it might be easier to modify the movement patterns of humans. Improved disease surveillance in healthy populations of wild and domestic animals and in groups of humans who are at elevated risk of infection will improve detection of disease outbreaks and allow authorities to more promptly begin disease transmission control actions. In every area, however, the benefits from improvements in response efficiency and effectiveness are of such magnitude that mitigation efforts should first be focused in this domain. As experience is gained in applying this risk assessment methodology, and concrete improvement steps are taken to reduce the risk of influenza transmission, preparedness for all communicable diseases will improve. This risk assessment process will become more accurate and relevant as more is learned about disease transmission patterns in specific areas and the value of various measures in controlling disease spread is determined.

Findings in the self-assessment process may illuminate routine practices that become a high-priority concern only when an infectious disease outbreak occurs. It is important that responsible authorities be aware of these practices and

> *Findings in the self-assessment process may illuminate routine practices that become a high priority concern only when an infectious disease outbreak occurs.*

---

[46] World Health Organization, "Responding to the Avian Influenza Pandemic Threat: Recommended Strategic Actions." Geneva: World Health Organization, 2005, WHO/CDS/CSR/GIP/2005.8). Available at: <http://www.who.int/csr/resources/publications/influenza/WHO_CDS_CSR_GIP_05_8-EN.pdf>, accessed October 23, 2005.

reasonable strategies for intervention so they can quickly react to these vulnerabilities when they suspect a disease outbreak. Examples of such practices in southeast China are rural-urban migration, intensive animal husbandry, slaughtering practices on village farms as well as in urban markets, and minimal hygiene standards. Scientists have long known about the closeness between man and animals in Guangdong Province and the presence of an ecosystem for the interaction of their common viruses.[47] Because of the sharing of influenza virus between ducks and chickens and the close proximity of humans, there has been speculation that the reassortment of genetic material between animal and human influenza viruses could occur in the animal reservoirs of these viruses.[48] Regular migration of people between rural areas and the large coastal cities of China facilitates the rapid spread of any potential new viruses in both directions. These factors are an integral part of demographic patterns and agricultural practices in China, and steps to change them during a period of low disease transmission risk would not be economically or socially feasible. During times of increased risk of infection, however, these practices may represent early opportunities to effectively intervene with selective movement and/or trade restrictions.

During the SARS outbreak, for example, Chinese officials recognized that *coronavirus* (the causative agent of SARS) transmission likely had occurred in open air wild animal markets in Guangdong Province. When isolated cases of SARS appeared in Guangdong the following year in January 2004, Guangdong authorities understood that despite the economic cost to market traders and animal breeders, the wild animal trade had to be stopped. The provincial government ordered a mass cull of civet cats, badgers, and raccoon dogs and a ban on their sale. These actions acted as a brake on one possible route of SARS viral transmission from animals to humans.[49]

An initial risk assessment methodology is presented below. While some of the factors presented may be more important than others, each is rated on a three-point scale of low risk, moderate risk, and high risk, and is assigned a score of zero, one, or two, respectively (there are a few exceptions where factors are assigned a score of either 0 or 2). Total scores serve to indicate the overall international infectious disease risk as low (fewer than 50 points), moderate (51–100 points), or high (more than 100 points). Users will note that multiple actions can be taken that, when considered in isolation, seem to have little overall effect but, when considered in aggregate, decrease disease transmission risk significantly. As this process is applied within countries and regions, a more accurate scoring methodology is likely to develop that improves its predictive precision, but the current process will allow agencies and authorities to gain familiarity with the risk factors and to take initial steps in self-assessment and disease transmission risk reduction. The steps in this process will be demonstrated more fully in the case study that follows.

---

[47] K.F. Shortridge and C.H. Stuart-Harris, "An Influenza Epicentre?" *Lancet* 320 (8302), October 1982, 812–813.

[48] Gabriel Leung, Anthony Hedley, Edith Lau and Tai-Hing Lam, "The Public Health Viewpoint," in Loh and Civic Exchange, eds., 58.

[49] Thomas Abraham, *Twenty-First Century Plague: The Story of SARS* (Baltimore: Johns Hopkins University Press, 2005), 131.

Step 1: Local Self-Assessment

The first step is based on multiple *ecological* (to include geographic, disease reservoir, population), *infrastructure*, and *response* factors that are widely recognized as contributing to disease transmission risk, such as exposure to an animal disease reservoir, person-to-person transmission characteristics, and the existence of the infrastructure to detect and respond to an infectious disease threat quickly. Multiple response factors are considered, which permits an objective assessment of the capabilities required to quickly detect and respond to an initial disease outbreak and to safely and effectively care for the infected cases. This self-assessment will provide a local baseline risk (LBR) score between 0 and 67, where a low score indicates low risk, and a high score indicates elevated risk. Responsible authorities may use the factors that make up the score to identify areas in which they should focus their mitigation efforts so they may improve their preparedness as efficiently as possible.

Step 1: Local Self-Assessment

Local <u>Baseline</u> Risk (LBR) = E + I + R

E = Ecological
I = Infrastructure
R = Response

Country-specific self-assessment factors allow determination of high-risk factors and identification of factors for <u>local</u> improvement.

Step 2: External Perceptions

The next step considers external perceptions of a country's internal preparedness and response capabilities. This can be accomplished in one of two ways. Either the country conducting the local self-assessment (step 1) can make an educated guess regarding another country's perception of its internal preparedness and response capabilities, or it can query the other side for an external assessment. Ideally, one would do both. The discrepancies between the two sources create an unprecedented opportunity for dialogue, for understanding the issues from differing points of view, for appreciating the other side's choices, as a means of reassessing one's own options for action, and for the kind of communication that can lead to cooperative as well as collaborative relationships. This assessment is not limited to countries; domestically, provinces or even adjoining townships could develop a similar mechanism to improve cooperation. These actions enjoy the further benefit of increasing the number of options available for risk reduction through cooperation and can lead to a more constructive strategy for dealing with risk reduction.

Assessing external perceptions is limited by the data available and thus is critically dependent on the degree of openness and information-sharing between two actors. Some may say that external perceptions of internal preparedness are irrelevant and should be ignored, but when international trust is adversely affected, with potentially detrimental actions and reactions in international travel, international trade, foreign direct investment, and stock value on international exchange markets, such perceptions become very important indeed.

The consideration and measurement of transparency factors is an important aspect of managing external perceptions. Many features of a country's governance play a role in openness and misunderstandings about internal priorities and conditions are common. In some countries and cultures, institutions may be more or less able to discuss infectious disease issues openly. Internal response capabilities may be a matter of some sensitivity, and bureaucratic coordination requirements that influence who may speak officially and unofficially may differ from country to country. But ultimately, differences in internal and external assessments of perceptions and the dialogue that can ensue do affect transparency.

The transparency factors used for international perceptions are more subjective than the preparedness and response factors, due to wide variations around the world. Some may debate the criteria used or the individual weights, but what is not debatable is that openness and transparency play a huge role in international perception. For this reason, the weight of the seven transparency factors described in the previous section is doubled when the international baseline risk (IBR) is calculated. This increases the range of the risk score to a high risk score of 95.

Step 2: External Perceptions

(Perceived) International Baseline Risk (IBR) = LBR + 2T

LBR = Local Baseline Risk
T = Transparency

Indicator of likely perception in international arena; highlights areas important for transparency.

Step 3: International Response

The most important factor to determine international disease transmission risk is the international response posture (IRP) score. While the LBR and IBR are specific to geography, ecology, population, infrastructure, and transparency, the IRP is based on disease-specific outbreak and transmission factors, and the presence of the particular disease anywhere in the world. This score represents a blending of the transmission characteristics of the disease agent with the likelihood of interrupting disease transmission in a particular geographic area. The score reflects the observation that the tipping point, that point where an infectious disease becomes an epidemic, varies with different disease pathogens and local capabilities to quickly control person-to-person transmission. A disease that is less communicable from person to person is less likely to reach the tipping point where it causes an epidemic than is a highly transmissible infection. On the other hand, a jurisdiction, state, or country that is less prepared for such an infectious disease event is more likely to reach this tipping point, quickly exhaust its resources, and experience breakdown in social structure than one that is better prepared.

45

The IRP score allows determination of the transmission risk for a specific disease by country and locality. This score will be constant for a disease where the animal reservoir, animal-to-human transmission characteristics, and person-to-person transmission mechanism is well known. It will be much more complex for an unknown pathogen, one in which transmission mechanisms are not fully understood, or when such transmission characteristics are undergoing change, such as HPAI A/H5N1 avian influenza.

The overall IRP is determined by multiplying the previously determined IBR by the disease outbreak transmission score. A factor is incorporated that takes into consideration the specific disease under investigation. For avian influenza, this factor works out to 0.063 in the current methodology. This factor takes into account the WHO Pandemic Alert Phases for avian influenza, but it will be different for other infectious diseases.

Step 3: International Response

International Response Posture (IRP) = IBR x 0.063DOT

IBR = International Baseline Risk
DOT = Disease Outbreak Transmission

Clarifies perceived country-specific risk to other countries—that is, *does this country pose more risk to others and therefore justifies more protective actions within my own country?* Such protective actions often lead to economic impacts related to travel, investment, and capital markets.

Step 4: Identify Areas for Intervention

Once scores have been calculated for steps 1 through 3, opportunities for intervention can be sought. First, factors that are assigned a high score should all be examined to determine if changes are both possible and practical. Areas that contributed to the elevated risk score but were not modified should be reexamined. Those that were determined to be impossible to modify should be considered as high-risk areas where additional disease surveillance or other types of monitoring might offer some degree of risk reduction, or at least early warning of an impending infectious disease outbreak. Other

> *...areas where modification or risk mitigation is determined to be impractical due to cost or other obstacles should be considered high-priority focus areas once a disease outbreak occurs.*

areas where modification or risk mitigation was determined to be impractical due to cost or other obstacles should be considered high-priority focus areas once a disease outbreak occurs. An action that may be impractical or difficult to implement under normal circumstances may become a viable option when emergency steps are being taken to control a raging epidemic.

In other words, producing a suite of possible responses may be impractical in advance of an outbreak because the relative costs and benefits may change once an outbreak occurs. If one has an appropriate tool, however, for assessing risk among the various factors provided by the methodology advanced in this paper, then decisionmakers will be able to broaden their repertoire of choices available to respond to a contingency and will be less likely to react rashly in the face of a potential crisis. For example, local economic agricultural factors may discourage widespread culling of exposed domestic chickens, limiting the culling only to those birds in an infected flock. Once an outbreak occurs, however, authorities may determine that the elevated risk does call for more widespread culling of populations within 3 kilometers of infected flocks. Domestic farmers may hide their small flocks from authorities because of the economic loss, but if reimbursement is raised to the point where farmers do not suffer great financial hardship, these farmers may come forward, increasing the effectiveness of efforts to interrupt transmission.

Step 5: Take Action

At this point, the actual mitigation steps should be taken to modify the area as appropriate to decrease the risk of infectious disease transmission. Important areas are early detection of an outbreak so effective actions may be taken, rapid characterization of the pathogen (including its reservoir and transmission characteristics and the clinical symptoms of diseases it causes), rapid and effective incident response, and open information-sharing with the public using print and broadcast media. Examples will be considered in more detail in the case study.

Step 6: Repeat Self-Assessment to Determine Effect of Interventions

The final step is to repeat the self-assessment after mitigation strategies have been applied to determine whether intervention efforts were adequate to decrease the level of risk. A decreased risk score will demonstrate that mitigation efforts are likely to have been effective in reducing disease transmission risks, but this repeat self-assessment should be performed by another person who was not directly involved in the interventions, so as candid an assessment as possible is achieved.

The next section provides a detailed case study focusing on avian influenza that demonstrates the use of the methodology described in this section, assessing the risk factors for a notional country and developing a prevention and risk mitigation strategy.

Avian Influenza Disease Transmission Risk Assessment Case Study

The risk of avian influenza A/H5N1 undergoing genetic reassortment, developing the ability for rapid person-to-person transmission, and causing a global influenza pandemic underscores the timeliness of this complex case study. The results demonstrate that the key elements that contribute to the tipping point include high traffic areas, disease surveillance systems that provide early detection of cases and assist with contact tracing, efficient coordination of prevention and response activities with other agencies and sectors, and open risk communication with the public about preventive measures that may be taken. As the reader works through the steps of the self-assessment, the utility of the risk mitigation process will become more apparent.

A notional Southeast Asian "country" is used to demonstrate the value of the self-assessment methodology for identifying and prioritizing preparation and mitigation opportunities. It does not represent a single country; rather, it represents characteristics of countries that could be at greatest risk (anywhere in the world) by virtue of their socioeconomic structure. The country used here is only placed in Southeast Asia to demonstrate the relationship among hot, warm, and cold zones, in the context where avian influenza and SARS have been most prevalent over the past few years. The self-assessment will be applied, opportunities for intervention will be prioritized, and then the self-assessment will be repeated to demonstrate the effect of the interventions.

This country has several large urban cities, shares several land borders with other countries, and has an ocean border. It has a rural population that is primarily involved in subsistence agriculture, a relatively underdeveloped public health infrastructure, and little government involvement in animal husbandry and agricultural practices. The healthcare delivery system is not advanced. As points of reference, the infant mortality rate is high at 77 deaths per 1,000 live births, the life expectancy at birth is 67 years, and the literacy rate is 68 percent. The country has a relatively closed press, there is no significant risk communication to the public, and the country does not report diseases to the WHO in a timely manner. No other details about governance are relevant to the basic risk assessment methodology.

What follows is intended to help the reader work through the risk assessment process by outlining the development of a risk assessment and mitigation strategy for avian influenza step by step. All choices are described fully in the questionnaires at Appendix A. Blank worksheets are available for use at Appendix B. Note that most items in the assessment that follows (with few exceptions) are based on survey questions ranked on a scale of zero to two.

Step 1: Local Self-Assessment

The local self-assessment was conducted using the description of risk assessment and mitigating factors and checklist in the appendix. For this notional Southeast Asian country, the checklist is completed in the following fashion.

ECOLOGICAL FACTORS WORKSHEET

(Choices and corresponding scores for Ecological Factors E-1 through E-6 are explained in the Appendix)

Factor	Score	Description
E-1	1	The country has a tropical climate.
E-2	2	The country is within 12 hours' travel by air from Vietnam and China, where cases of avian influenza and SARS have been present in recent years.
E-3	1	The country is within 48 hours of Vietnam and China by truck or ship.
E-4	2	The country has several large urban cities.
E-5	2	The country has a busy international airport and several very busy border crossings.
E-6	2	The country has vulnerable children, pregnant women, and elderly in both urban and rural impoverished settings.

TOTAL Ecological Factors Score: 10

INFRASTRUCTURE FACTORS WORKSHEET

(Choices and corresponding scores for Infrastructure Factors I-1 through I-9 are explained in the Appendix)

Factor	Score	Description
I-1	2	There are large numbers of backyard farms where chickens, ducks, pigs, and people come into close contact.
I-2	2	The public health disease surveillance system is ineffective.
I-3	1	The rural population is largely dispersed and is difficult to reach quickly.
I-4	2	The public health system is inadequate to investigate and diagnose a disease outbreak and to effectively interrupt disease transmission. External assistance would be required if an outbreak were to occur.
I-5	2	Clinical and laboratory diagnostics are very limited, requiring clinical samples to be sent out to WHO reference laboratories.
I-6	2	The healthcare delivery system is relatively underdeveloped. Medical supply and equipment shortages are common and healthcare personnel availability gaps exist.
I-7	2	Hospitals are limited to basic infection control practices.
I-8	2	Risk communication with the public is not practiced.
I-9	2	Communication and coordination between government agencies is limited at the national and regional levels.

TOTAL Infrastructure Factors Score: 17

RESPONSE FACTORS WORKSHEET

(Choices and corresponding scores for Response Factors R-1 through R-19 are explained in the Appendix)

Factor	Score	Description
R-1	2	Animal and human health officials are not involved in any disease prevention activities.
R-2	2	The public health system is not developed; human health officials are not involved in any disease prevention activities.
R-3	2	Human health officials are not involved in any disease prevention activities.
R-4	2	There are no risk communication activities in response to disease outbreaks.
R-5	2	Animal health officials are not involved in any disease surveillance activities.
R-6	2	Animal health officials are not involved in any disease prevention activities.
R-7	2	Animal health officials are not involved in any disease prevention activities.
R-8	2	Animal health officials are not involved in any disease prevention activities.
R-9	2	Animal health officials are not involved in any disease prevention activities.
R-10	2	Human health officials are not involved in any disease surveillance activities.
R-11	2	Human health officials are not involved in any disease surveillance activities.
R-12	2	Human health officials are not involved in any disease surveillance activities.
R-13	2	Human health officials are not involved in any disease surveillance activities.
R-14	2	Human health officials are not involved in any disease prevention activities.
R-15	2	Human health officials are not involved in any disease prevention activities.
R-16	2	The healthcare system provides only basic clinical care; public health officials do not interact with clinicians to emphasize infectious precautions and notification of potentially infectious cases.
R-17	2	Laboratory diagnostics are limited to basic services only.
R-18	1	Healthcare services are limited to those with sufficient money and prestige.
R-19	2	Interagency response coordination does not occur.

TOTAL Response Factors Score: 37

After completing the ecological, infrastructure and response factors sections, the total local baseline risk score is obtained by adding the ecological, infrastructure, and response totals:

$$\text{Total Local Baseline Risk (LBR)} =$$
$$\text{Ecological + Infrastructure + Response} =$$
$$10 + 17 + 37 = 64$$

This local baseline risk score is based on self-assessment, and is one of the highest risk scores that can be achieved in this current methodology, where 67 is the highest score possible. At this point in the self-assessment, it becomes apparent that many areas that raise the risk for communicable disease transmission in this country exist. These areas will be examined in detail in step 4.

Step 2: External Perceptions

The next step is to consider transparency factors, so that authorities in the country conducting the assessment can determine how external actors—nations and others—are likely to perceive the risk of an infectious disease spreading internationally.

Step 2: External Perceptions

TRANSPARENCY FACTORS WORKSHEET

(Choices and corresponding scores for Transparency Factors T-1 through T-7 are explained in the Appendix)

Factor	Score	Description
T-1	2	Historically, containment efforts have been ineffective for communicable diseases, requiring external assistance from other countries and multilateral organizations to organize the investigation, manage the health consequences, and identify protective measures to reduce future vulnerability.
T-2	1	Historically, previous communicable disease outbreaks have led to partial disruptions of essential public services, both directly by disease cases appearing in those who work in these sectors and indirectly from people fleeing the area in fear to avoid exposure.
T-3	2	No information about strengths and weaknesses of the public health system is released by government authorities, nor is any proactive risk communication done about disease outbreaks or protective steps that can be taken.
T-4	2	No information is released about cases of disease during an actual outbreak.
T-5	2	There is little evidence of public trust in the governing authorities. There have been periodic uses of force in the past to control dissent.
T-6	2	Media outlets are controlled by the government and do not report any information that may be deemed unfavorable.
T-7	2	Disease outbreaks are reported to the World Health Organization months after they have been brought under control; numbers of cases are felt to be underestimated.

TOTAL Transparency Factors Score: 13

The total international baseline risk score is then derived by adding the local baseline risk to the transparency factors score multiplied by two:

$$\textbf{Total International Baseline Risk (IBR) =}$$
$$\textbf{Local Baseline Risk + 2 x Transparency =}$$
$$\textbf{64 + 2(13) = 90}$$

This international baseline risk score is also one of the highest risk scores that can be achieved in this current methodology, in which 95 is the highest score possible.

At this point in the self-assessment, results indicate that this country is perceived to be at very high disease transmission risk on the international stage. The difference between the local baseline risk and the international baseline risk is striking, in that the lack of external visibility about internal infrastructure and response capabilities causes external actors to assume the worst about the nation's communicable disease risk. Actions that are taken by other countries will be based on this very high international baseline risk score of 90, rather than the high local baseline risk score of 64.

Step 3: International Response

The third step in the self-assessment is to determine the degree of risk for international spread by reevaluating the disease transmission risk based on the particular disease or pathogen of concern. This portion of the self-assessment is more complex for avian influenza than for many other infectious agents, since risk must be considered for each of the six WHO pandemic phases described in Section 4.

The next worksheet summarizes the risk score for each disease-specific outbreak and transmission (DOT) factor for each of the WHO pandemic phases for avian influenza. It is used to determine the degree of risk for international spread of the disease pathogen, avian influenza.

DISEASE-SPECIFIC OUTBREAK AND TRANSMISSION (DOT) FACTORS

(Choices and corresponding scores for DOT Factors DOT-1 through DOT-18 are explained in the Appendix)

Factor	Description	WHO Phases					
		1	2	3	4	5	6
DOT-1	Disease endemic in the geographic area	0	2	2	2	2	2
DOT-2	Disease is caused by unknown agent, unusual transmission	0	0	0	1	2	2
DOT-3	Disease caused by environmental pathogen	1	2	2	2	2	2
DOT-4	Animal reservoir for the disease	1	1	1	2	2	2
DOT-5	Animal reservoir highly mobile	1	1	1	1	1	1
DOT-6	Transmission between different types of reservoir animals	2	2	2	2	2	2
DOT-7	Mixing between wild and domestic animals	2	2	2	2	2	2
DOT-8	Animal-to-human transmission of disease	0	1	1	1	2	2
DOT-9	Person-to-person transmission of disease	0	0	0	1	2	2
DOT-10	Disease pathogenicity in animal reservoir	2	2	2	2	2	2
DOT-11	Disease pathogenicity in humans	1	2	2	2	2	2
DOT-12	Unusual disease occurrence for area, season, population	0	0	0	0	2	2
DOT-13	More severe evolution of cases or unusual symptoms	0	0	0	1	2	2
DOT-14	Disease occurs in area of high international traffic	0	0	0	0	2	2
DOT-15	Disease occurs in area of limited sanitary control	1	1	1	1	2	2
DOT-16	Increased mobility of high-risk groups	0	0	0	2	2	2
DOT-17	Disease cases develop among healthcare personnel	0	0	0	1	2	2
DOT-18	Initial disease case has high-risk travel or exposure history	0	0	0	1	2	2
TOTAL Disease Outbreak and Transmission Factors Scores		11	16	16	22	35	35

By way of brief analysis, the following table provides the rationale the authors used to assign values to each DOT factor above.

	DISEASE-SPECIFIC OUTBREAK AND TRANSMISSION FACTORS ANALYSIS		
Factor	**Self-Assessment of International Response**		
DOT-1	According to WHO definitions, once there is an animal influenza subtype circulating with substantial risk of human disease, the world is in phase 2. All countries or geographic regions where this virus is present have a risk score of 2 from phase 2 through phase 6.		
DOT-2	The risk score increases from 0 to 2 as the virus moves from its animal reservoir into humans despite all control measures. This takes place between phase 3 and phase 5. It is reasonable to assume that the virus is becoming more adapted to humans at this point.		
DOT-3	The lowest risk score for this factor is 1, since avian influenza is by definition a pathogen of birds. As soon as the virus is circulating and is felt to be a risk to humans, the risk score becomes 2. This occurs early, at phase 2.		
DOT-4	When present, avian influenza may infect domestic chickens or ducks, other domestic birds or those kept as pets, or a variety of wild birds. HPAI A/H5N1 may be spreading globally by migratory waterfowl, and so appears to be impossble to eradicate. Viral outbreaks in domestic birds in an area where they can be quickly culled would justify a risk score of 1, but the current global spread by migratory waterfowl will likely disseminate this viral strain globally. Retrospective analysis after the virus has spread into wild bird populations around the world may suggest that this factor should be scored in a different fashion. Other mechanisms for global spread may exist.		
DOT-5	The risk score for this factor remains at 1 for all WHO phases, since there are no particular bird species that are highly adapted to manmade conveyance.		
DOT-6	The current HPAI A/H5N1 appears to be freely transmitted between different species of birds, swine, felids, and rodents. The risk score is 2 across all WHO pandemic phases.		
DOT-7	The current HPAI A/H5N1 appears to be freely transmitted between wild and domestic birds. The risk score is 2 across all WHO pandemic phases.		
DOT-8	This factor coincides directly with the WHO pandemic phases. The risk score elevates from 0 to 1 between phase 1 and 2, and from 1 to 2 when the virus becomes more adapted to humans between phases 5 and 6.		
DOT-9	Person-to-person transmission begins at phase 4 with a risk score of 1, and increases at phase 5 with a risk score of 2.		
DOT-10	HPAI A/H5N1 is highly pathogenic in chickens and in some wild waterfowl, but appears to cause subclinical illness in some ducks and perhaps other species. The risk score is assumed to be 2 in all phases for the sake of discussion, though this may change as viral characteristics are further understood.		
DOT-11	Disease pathogenicity in humans appears to be high as of the end of 2005, but the discovery of serologic evidence of human disease in Turkey without clinical symptoms may call for the current score of 2 to be changed as the virus is characterized further.		
DOT-12	This factor is difficult in the case of HPAI A/H5N1, since so little is currently known about the virus, its reservoir, and its clinical symptoms. For the sake of this discussion, the risk score is 0 until the virus becomes more adaptable to humans in phase 5. As the clinical and epidemiological characteristics are described, some may choose to attribute a score of 0 or 2 across all phases.		
DOT-13	This factor is also dependent on further characterization of the clinical symptoms and course of disease. Risk scores increase in this case study as viral transmission characteristics defy control efforts.		
DOT-14	Successful isolation and control of human cases through phase 4 limits the risk score to 0. Unsuccessful transmission control in phase 5 raises the risk score to 2.		

DOT-15	A risk score of 1 is the best possible in this notional southeast Asian country, given its underdeveloped public health system and high burden of disease. The risk score increases to 2 when person-to-person transmission increases in phase 5.
DOT-16	The risk scores for this factor parallel that seen for SARS in Asia, where agricultural and healthcare worker mobility led to community transmission. The risk score increases from 0 to 2 when human transmissibility increases in phase 5.
DOT-17	As in factor 16 above, the risk scores parallel the SARS experience. Increased human transmissibility puts healthcare workers, and the healthcare system, at greater risk, so the risk scores increase in phases 4 through 6.
DOT-18	The risk score for this factor is greatly dependent on the initial case or cases. The scores in this case study increase from phases 4 through 6 due to the underdeveloped public health system in this country and the inability to perform prompt, effective contact tracing. Lower scores would be appropriate for a country with a more robust local and regional public health system.

This third step of the assessment may be the most complex, as many of the risk factors depend on information not yet available, such as animal-to-animal transmission, global animal movement, animal-to-human transmission, and person-to-person transmission. The most important practical application, though, is to perform this self-assessment based on the information available, so that mitigation changes can be started. The detailed scientific and clinical information that will become available over time will have little direct impact on which improvement steps should be taken.

Careful consideration of the WHO pandemic phases and the associated public health goals for each phase reveals that actual human disease containment actions do not begin until phase 4. The goals for phases 1 through 3 focus on preparedness, improving surveillance systems, and viral characterization. This risk assessment methodology reflects these priorities, where the international response posture score remains essentially the same as the international baseline risk score through phase 3. Once active person-to-person transmission begins in phase 4, however, risk for international disease transmission increases, resulting in a significantly elevated risk posed by an unprepared country to other countries. Steps taken by other countries should reflect this increased risk.

The international response posture is derived by multiplying the international baseline risk score by 0.063 times the DOT factor for the particular WHO pandemic phase. The factor 0.063 is used to keep the effects of the DOT factors from affecting the risk score until there is known person-to-person transmission of avian influenza. A different factor must be derived as this risk assessment methodology is adapted to other contagious diseases.

The international response posture score for the notional Southeast Asian country during WHO pandemic phase 3 is 91 (90.72 is rounded up to the nearest whole number).

International Response Posture (IRP) =
International Baseline Risk (IBR) x 0.063 x Total DOT Factor (WHO Phase 3)
90 x 0.063 x 16 = 90.72 → 91

It is essentially the same risk score as the international baseline risk score of 90. When active person-to-person transmission begins and the WHO raises the alert level to phase 4, the score increases to 125. Lack of presence of avian influenza in a particular country would offer a degree of reassurance to other countries, but in a location such as this notional Southeast Asian country, the absence of evidence of the virus is not reassuring, since baseline animal and human disease surveillance systems are insufficient and may not be able to detect an outbreak in a timely manner.

Step 4: Identify Areas for Intervention

Mitigation steps are taken based on the degree of risk and the feasibility of making changes. With respect to HPAI A/H5N1, these intervention opportunities should be identified according to areas of highest vulnerability; areas where interventions are likely to be practical; and areas where interventions will be most likely to decrease the risk score.

First, as described in Section 2, *detection of the outbreak in its earliest stages is critical, so effective actions may be started*. Detection requires distinguishing actual cases from the usual background noise of an animal or human disease surveillance system; therefore, the improvement of surveillance systems is often an essential aspect of risk mitigation. Authorities in many areas of the world under-invest in animal and human disease surveillance systems, erroneously assuming that they will learn about such disease cases when enough of them develop to be noticed by the general public or by medical personnel who treat these diseases. This fallacious belief overlooks the importance of early intervention to contain a disease outbreak, as is apparent by the risk scores in this methodology. Developing new animal and human disease surveillance systems and enhancing existing ones are the most appropriate first steps to communicable disease transmission risk reduction.

> **...detection of the outbreak in its earliest stages is critical, so effective actions may be started.**

Second, *rapid characterization of the pathogen, including its reservoir and transmission characteristics and the clinical syndrome it causes, is essential so that scarce medical treatment resources may be applied where most indicated*. The risk assessment methodology points to the importance of understanding these characteristics, as the risk score increases when these characteristics are unknown. This suggests that intervention efforts (such as rapid and complete epidemiological investigations, contact tracing, and rapid laboratory verification of pathogen strains) that provide such information as quickly as possible will reduce overall risk.

Third, a *response is most likely to be effective when it is rapid and complete*. This requires each party to quickly take the correct action as described in the discussion about crisis phases so coordinated decisions across different response sectors lead to focused actions. These steps include prompt initial response by all response sectors, immediate data collection to accurately characterize the scope of the incident, and rapid notification of all other agencies that are likely to be involved in a comprehensive response. Unique challenges exist when interagency coordination and cooperation is sought. These issues must be identified and considered early in the process of working across agencies, and policies developed as processes, procedures, and solutions are tested and refined. Two-way information-sharing must occur rapidly between different response agencies so actions can be coordinated appropriately. Processes and procedures may need to be developed so the elements of an effective response can be enacted; such processes should be tested in realistic exercises to ensure their adequacy.

Finally, *information-sharing must occur with the public using both print and broadcast media.* Instructions should be provided on steps that can be taken to avoid exposure, such as avoidance of chickens and other birds that appear ill, careful hand washing after contact with potentially contaminated produce, and thorough cooking of poultry products. Symptoms of influenza and instructions for seeking medical attention should be described in language understood by the entire population. Healthcare workers should be notified about personal protective measures and the importance of prompt reporting of suspected cases to public health authorities. Once an outbreak occurs, the public should be informed of the behavior needed to prevent further exposure and of any community-wide steps being taken to prevent disease transmission, such as social distancing.

Step 5: Take Action

The first priority area identified in step 4 is to *improve early detection with better animal and human disease surveillance*. Surveillance is the process of systematic collection, collation, and analysis of data, and its prompt dissemination to the appropriate authorities for relevant action to be taken. A well-functioning disease surveillance system provides information for planning, implementation, and monitoring and evaluation of public health intervention programs.[50]

At a minimum, four steps should be taken to implement an *animal disease surveillance system*. The first step is to identify the diseases of interest (in this case study, avian influenza). Second, priority areas where disease surveillance should take place must be identified. For avian influenza, this should include areas where migratory waterfowl are found, commercial poultry production facilities, areas in the community where poultry are produced in backyards, and markets where live poultry are sold. Third, reporting responsibilities of farmers, animal health workers, veterinarians, and other agricultural officials must be identified. Finally, data collection processes, including the thresholds at which various disease findings will trigger specific actions, must be identified. These processes are described in greater detail by the FAO *Manual on Livestock Disease Surveillance and Information Systems*.[51] Actions to minimize transmission should be taken, such as culling infected and exposed animals.

Human disease surveillance begins with identifying febrile respiratory diseases that could be caused by influenza, using both clinical symptoms to focus on those persons with respiratory illnesses most likely to be influenza and laboratory tests to determine if H5N1 or another influenza serotype is the cause of the illness. Most public health systems use sentinel sites that are representative of various geographic areas to act as early warning indicators that influenza may be present in an area.[52] Cases are initially identified using a specific case definition (fever over 38°C, and cough or sore throat in the absence of other diagnoses). Laboratory confirmation is necessary for epidemiological investigation, either by virus isolation, detection of influenza virus antigen, or by fourfold increase in antibody titer on early and late sera. Cases are often reported weekly from such sentinel sites.

---

[50] World Health Organization, "Protocol for the Assessment of National Communicable Disease Surveillance and Response Systems: Guidelines for Assessment Teams," WHO/CDS/CSR/ISR/2001.2, 2001. Available at: <http://www.who.int/csr/resources/publications/surveillance/whocdscsrisr20012.pdf>, accessed January 18, 2006.
[51] United Nations Food and Agriculture Organization, *Manual on Livestock Disease Surveillance and Information Systems*, 1999. Available at: <http://www.fao.org/DOCREP/004/X3331E/X3331E01 htm#ch8>, accessed January 18, 2006.
[52] Toronto Public Health, "Toronto Pandemic Influenza Plan," November 2005. Available at: <http://www.toronto.ca/health/pandemicflu/>, accessed January 18, 2006.

Detailed descriptions of surveillance systems are available in the *WHO Recommended Surveillance Standards*.[53]

These animal and human disease surveillance systems should be coordinated so that both animal and human disease case finding improves in geographic areas where animal outbreaks are suspected or confirmed. For example, human disease reporting frequency may be increased from weekly to daily, the number of sentinel sites might be increased, or all physicians and hospitals might be asked to report every patient who might meet a certain case definition. The importance of integration between animal and human disease surveillance systems (including wildlife) cannot be sufficiently emphasized. Both avian influenza and SARS offer numerous examples of cases where such lack of integration has resulted in missed opportunities and failure to contain or control these diseases as quickly as they might have been.[54]

The second priority area is *rapid characterization of the pathogen and its reservoir, transmission characteristics, and the clinical syndromes it causes*. These actions build upon the animal and human surveillance systems described above and require prompt investigation of animal and human cases. For avian influenza, animal health experts and veterinarians should quickly identify the causes of unexpected animal deaths and attempt to determine the prevalence of asymptomatic disease in animal populations that are suspected of harboring the virus. Humans who may have come into contact with animals that are known or suspected to be infected with HPAI A/H5N1 should be carefully monitored for signs of clinical disease. Serology tests may be performed on those with respiratory symptoms to quickly determine the causative pathogens. Steps should be taken to separate domestic animals from wild animals if disease transmission is likely to occur in this manner. If any person-to-person transmission occurs or is suspected, complete contact tracing should be done promptly on any confirmed cases so those exposed can be isolated and monitored for the development of disease. If HPAI A/H5N1 is identified, prompt molecular fingerprinting should be performed so that transmission dynamics can be completely defined. Results of all these findings should be rapidly communicated to disease control and healthcare workers so detection and response practices may be improved. International coordinating bodies such as the WHO should quickly be notified so similar international alerts may be released.

The third priority area is a *rapid, coordinated response to animal and human cases*. The development of such a cross-jurisdictional response should begin with preparedness planning at all levels, as described in Section 2 on prevention phases. Practical steps that can be taken at the local, district, and provincial levels to develop such a coordinated initial response are:

- assembling a multidisciplinary planning committee
- reviewing applicable documents, plans, laws, and regulations
- performing vulnerability analysis to identify weaknesses
- evaluating system capability and capacity to respond
- identifying necessary tasks and requirements

---

[53] World Health Organization, *WHO Recommended Surveillance Standards, 2nd Edition*, WHO/CDS/CSR/ISR/99.2, 1999. Available at: <http://www.who.int/csr/resources/publications/surveillance/whocdscsrisr992.pdf>, accessed January 18, 2006.
[54] For a particularly well-written piece on this subject, see T. Kuiken et al., "Pathogen Surveillance in Animals," *Science*, Vol. 309, September 9, 2005, 1680–1681.

- matching capabilities and capacities to requirements
- enhancing system capabilities and capacity
- developing plans, techniques, tactics, and procedures
- implementing education, training, and exercise opportunities
- establishing a continuous preparedness improvement program

Integrated interagency response requires that specific coordination and cooperation challenges be considered. Some of these challenges are:

- international, national, regional, state, local (terms may vary from country to country)
- communications—routine and crisis
- incident command
    o Who is in charge?
    o When does responsibility shift, and how is this accomplished?
- overlapping roles and responsibilities
- funding and reimbursement
- communication with the public
- coordination between agencies
- development of interagency policies

As these aspects of interagency interaction are developed and tested, communication and coordination processes can be developed and implemented so that responses to an outbreak can take place quickly and efficiently.

Public messages should be developed about steps to be taken at different points in an outbreak and should be made available in as many languages and through all media necessary to reach as many sectors of society as possible. Spokespersons should be identified for each relevant agency and response sector, and opinion leaders should be identified and involved in the planning for communication of these public safety messages. Members of broadcast and print media agencies should be educated about the types of messages that will be provided and the anticipated schedule of daily information briefings during an emergency response. Points of contact should be provided for any interviews that may be desired before and during a response.

Step 6: Repeat Self-Assessment to Determine Effect of Interventions

The final step is to repeat the self-assessment after mitigation strategies have been applied to determine whether intervention efforts were adequate to decrease the level of risk. The pre- and post-assessment scores are filled out in the next worksheet.

POST-ASSESSMENT WORKSHEET

FACTOR	SCORE		COMMENT
	Pre-	Post-	

Ecological Factors—No change possible

Infrastructure Factors—Decrease from 17 to 13

FACTOR	Pre-	Post-	COMMENT
I-1	2	2	No change.
I-2	2	1	The public health disease surveillance system is improved somewhat.
I-3	1	1	No change.
I-4	2	2	No change.
I-5	2	1	Clinical and laboratory diagnostics are improved with rapid influenza diagnostics.
I-6	2	2	No change.
I-7	2	2	No change.
I-8	2	1	Basic risk communication processes. Procedures and messages are developed.
I-9	2	1	Communication and coordination between government agencies is begun.

Response Factors—Decrease from 37 to 17

FACTOR	Pre-	Post-	COMMENT
R-1	2	0	Animal reservoirs identified.
R-2	2	0	Disease transmission risk factors identified.
R-3	2	0	High-risk groups identified.
R-4	2	1	Public risk communication activities beginning.
R-5	2	1	Animal disease surveillance beginning.
R-6	2	1	Animal health officials beginning to take steps to protect animals from disease.
R-7	2	1	Steps taken to separate domestic animals from wild animals when disease cases detected in geographic region.
R-8	2	1	Animal health officials take partial steps to cull infected animal populations.
R-9	2	1	Animal health officials take partial steps to cull exposed animal populations.

R-10	2	1	Basic human disease surveillance processes are begun.
R-11	2	1	Human health officials attempt to implement disease surveillance in high-risk areas such as airports and border crossings.
R-12	2	2	Insufficient enhancement of surveillance processes to determine pathogenicity.
R-13	2	1	Human case finding is improved by encouraging case reporting.
R-14	2	1	Contact tracing is begun on high-risk exposure groups.
R-15	2	1	Public messages encourage exposed persons to seek medical attention.
R-16	2	1	Voluntary isolation of infected persons is encouraged.
R-17	2	1	Improved laboratory diagnostic capability is developed in referral hospitals.
R-18	1	1	Healthcare services are limited to those with sufficient money and prestige.
R-19	2	1	Interagency response coordination efforts are started.

Transparency Factors—Decrease from 13 to 7

T-1	2	1	Disease containment efforts improved, partially due to internal capacity building and partially to prompt requests for external assistance from multilateral organizations.
T-2	1	1	Interventions are not sufficient to impact effects of a disease outbreak on public infrastructure.
T-3	2	1	Government authorities provide information about risk factors for disease outbreaks and steps that are being taken to improve response capabilities.
T-4	2	1	Government authorities provide limited information about disease outbreaks and control measures.
T-5	2	1	Governing authorities tolerate mild criticism of lack of preparedness in the press and acknowledge that improvements are necessary and under way.
T-6	2	1	Media outlets are permitted to report accurate information about disease outbreaks and government intervention efforts.
T-7	2	1	Disease outbreaks are reported to the World Health Organization weekly.

Post-Intervention Self-Assessment Results	Pre-	Post-
Local Baseline Risk (LBR)	64	40
International Baseline Risk (IBR)	90	54
International Response Posture (WHO Pandemic Phase 3)	91	54

TOTAL SCORES GUIDE: LOW=<50   MODERATE=51-100   HIGH=>100

This case study is designed to demonstrate the practicality of the risk assessment and mitigation methodology. The risk scores assigned to each risk factor are intended to show how system-wide risk assessment can direct interventions so that efforts may be applied to those aspects of the system that are most vulnerable and most likely to benefit. While minimal benefit may be derived from a focus on one or two of these steps, broad-based efforts are expected to yield significant improvements.

This intervention exercise contains many artificialities and assumptions but demonstrates effectively that disease transmission risks can be significantly reduced by way of relatively inexpensive interventions. The majority of these intervention steps depend on communication and coordination within and between sectors of the government. The degree of actual required training is minimal and well within reach of most nations and governments. Donor organizations can use this methodology to identify those efforts most likely to yield real improvement.

In this particular case study, the highlighted interventions did not completely eliminate the risk attributed to each particular area. As authorities continue to focus on the agriculture, healthcare, and public health systems, further risk reduction can take place.

Section Six
Conclusion

When lives are at stake, it is better to err on the side of overreaction than underreaction.[55] Public safety is maximized when decisions and potential outcomes are carefully considered before lives are at stake in a crisis setting. This paper presents an initial effort at understanding and managing the very complex biological, sociocultural, ecological, and political interactions centered on an international communicable disease outbreak so that crucial decisions can be considered now. While experts in each of these fields of study have contributed much to understanding the interaction of pathogen, environment, and host, and to the behavioral dimensions of people in their occupational and family settings, little is known about how individuals or populations respond in the face of an infectious disease threat. The realities of globalization, and the greater interaction among people

> *Public safety is maximized when decisions and potential outcomes are carefully considered before lives are at stake in a crisis setting.*

of different cultures as geographic barriers have fallen in recent decades, thrust decisionmakers at all levels of government into the uncomfortable position of facing global infectious disease threats with few if any additional tools and resources to utilize as they attempt to meet their public responsibilities. The self-assessment methodology presented in this paper begins to fill this void.

Disaster experts are considering methods to improve disaster response by in-depth analysis of all elements that may be contributory. Guidelines have been developed elsewhere for the study and evaluation of disasters, specifically from the perspective of medical effectiveness, efficacy, and cost-benefit relationships of disaster medical responses and relief efforts. Functional phases for the purpose of an academic model include the pre-event status as a point of reference, the actual event and its impact using a damage assessment, a needs assessment and various response options, changes in the health status of the affected population, and the restoration of this health status to its pre-event level.[56] The functional phases from these guidelines are being integrated into the Haddon matrix, a conceptual framework developed in the 1970s to help apply the science of epidemiology to practical injury prevention.[57] The integration of the Haddon matrix with these functional phases is likely to help disaster experts identify the factors that contribute to an injury before, during, and after an event occurs. A modified Haddon matrix has been created to consider the risk factors contributing to the 2005 London bombings.[58] As disaster science improves in the future, the risk factors described in this guide to management of an international contagious disease outbreak should be examined in the context of the Haddon matrix. Unanticipated factors thus may be

---

[55] David J. Sencer and J. Donald Millar, "Reflections on the 1976 Swine Flu Vaccination Program," *Emerging Infectious Diseases* 12, no. 1 (January 2006), 29–33.

[56] Task Force on Quality Control of Disaster Management, Knut Sundnes and Marvin Birnbaum, eds., "Health Disaster Management: Guidelines for Evaluation and Research in the Utstein Style," *Prehospital and Disaster Medicine* 17, supplement 3, 2003. Available at: <http://pdm.medicine.wisc.edu/Guidelines/TOCVol1.htm>, accessed January 2, 2006.

[57] Carol Runyan, "Introduction: Back to the Future—Revisiting Haddon's Conceptualization of Injury Epidemiology and Prevention," *Epidemiologic Reviews* 25, no. 1, 2003, 60–64.

[58] Jeffrey Arnold, "The 2005 London Bombings and the Haddon Matrix," *Prehospital and Disaster Medicine* 20, no. 5 2005, 278–281.

identified that have a significant effect on reducing the risk of an infectious disease outbreak, controlling its transmission, or restoring confidence in government.

The communicable disease risk assessment methodology described in this paper provides several essential starting points in preparedness, prevention, and education. Descriptions of various factors that contribute to disease transmission risk allow the user to identify local factors in the context of their day-to-day responsibilities, reduce risk where possible, and understand the initial steps to take as an emergency unfolds to minimize the risk of further spread. The importance of various infrastructure and response factors allows senior leaders and donor organizations to identify those areas where mitigation efforts are most likely to effectively reduce disease transmission risk. Finally, a common understanding of local and national risks, preparedness levels, and useful response steps facilitates a coordinated international response and reduces the likelihood of deterioration into a crisis. The value of this methodology lies in the fact that one can clearly identify factors that matter in thinking about assessment. The authors recognize that the quantitative scales provided in the worksheet will benefit from refinement, a future step that will be taken to improve the tool.

Internationally, communicable disease risk assessment and risk management are separate functions. While the WHO makes risk assessments and annual influenza vaccine recommendations, national authorities must choose how to accept, incorporate, and act upon such a global risk assessment. Risk management, on the other hand, involves taking steps to mitigate risk at the local level, and is the exclusive responsibility of governmental authorities, performed and funded by federal, state, central, provincial, or other governments as appropriate. Pandemic risk management, itself an uncertain art, must independently weigh ongoing risk assessment findings in the context of actions that best serve national and international interests.[59] This tool enables authorities to take practical steps to begin this risk assessment process. It also lays the foundation for creating a common lexicon and methodology to evaluate risk, take preventive action, enhance veterinary and medical cooperation in a way that improves the ability of governments to think and act strategically, and respond to a communicable disease outbreak in a way that is conducive to communication, collaboration, and cooperation to bridge gaps that no one country alone can do.

---

[59] Walter R. Dowdle, "Influenza Pandemic Periodicity, Virus Recycling, and the Art of Risk Assessment," *Emerging Infectious Diseases* 12, no. 1, January 2006, 34–39.

Appendix A
Risk Assessment and Mitigation Factors Questionnaire

- *Ecological Factors*

- *Infrastructure Factors*

- *Response Factors*

- *Transparency Factors*

- *Disease-Specific Outbreak and Transmission Factors*

Ecological Factors Questionnaire
(Score: 0–11)

Risk Assessment and Mitigation Factor   **Risk Score**

E-1. Environmental or biological conditions favorable to disease transmission

Tropical climates provide temperature and humidity that are more favorable to disease transmission than arid or temperate climates.

1 – Yes
0 – No

E-2. Travel links with countries with recent outbreaks of infectious diseases

Rapid air transit permits persons to travel from a high-risk country while incubating an infectious disease and makes movement restrictions more difficult to use to control disease transmission.

2 – Persons can enter the country within 12 hours of departing from a country at high risk of the infectious disease
1 – Persons can enter the country within 24 hours of departing from a country at high risk of the infectious disease
0 – Travel from a high-risk country requires more than 24 hours

E-3. Trade links with countries with recent outbreaks of infectious diseases

Movement of goods minimally increases risk of disease transmission (exception is by stowaway person or animal)

2 – Goods can enter the country within 24 hours of departure from a country at high risk of the infectious disease
1 – Goods can enter the country within 48 hours of departure from a country at high risk of the infectious disease
0 – Goods are in transit over 48 hours after departure from a country at high risk of the infectious disease

E-4. High degree of human interaction

Person-to-person transmission increases when humans are in close proximity.

2 – Urban environment
1 – Suburban
0 – Rural

E-5. High degree of population mobility

Increased movement leads to increased potential for exposure of large numbers of people and increased risk of disease transmission prior to identification of infected cases.

2 – High traffic volume (international airport, border crossing, urban mass transit)
1 – Moderate traffic volume (urban setting)
0 – Little to no population movement (rural setting)

69

E-6. Immunosuppressed populations at risk for the disease

Children, pregnant women, persons with HIV/AIDS. the elderly, and the severely malnourished are more susceptible to disease and would likely experience an increased death rate.

2 – Vulnerable children, pregnant women, persons with HIV/AIDS, the elderly, or severely
    malnourished populations are at high risk for exposure and unlikely to have early access to
    healthcare services
1 – Such populations present but with good access to healthcare services
0 – No vulnerable populations at risk

Total Ecological Factor Score: Range 0–11

70

Infrastructure Factors Questionnaire
(Score: 0–18)

Risk Mitigation and Assessment Factor   **Risk Score**

I-1. Presence of animal-human interaction

Risk for transmission of disease from animal reservoir to humans increases as contact increases.

2 – Domestic occupational contact between potential animal reservoirs and humans (i.e., backyard farms)
1 – Commercial occupational contact between potential animal reservoirs and humans (commercial animal production) or in hunting activities
0 – No regular animal-human contact

I-2. Effective human disease surveillance process

Prompt collection and reporting of diseases is necessary to direct disease investigation and control efforts.

2 – Disease surveillance and reporting nonexistent
1 – Disease surveillance and reporting functions only when special emphasis
0 – Well-developed disease surveillance and reporting process

I-3. Social, climate, or geographic response barriers

War, natural disaster, adverse weather conditions, geographically dispersed population would increase the difficulty in reaching needy populations.

2 – Uncertain social or climatic factors preventing response effectiveness (war, impassable weather)
1 – Geographic features present that decrease response effectiveness (dispersed populations, disrupted road, rail lines)
0 – No adverse factors that would hinder a response

I-4. External assistance needed to detect, investigate, respond to, and control disease or prevent new cases

Disease spread may occur before external assistance is available; healthcare infrastructure may be inadequate to treat cases.

2 – External disease investigation and treatment resources needed to respond to and manage outbreak
1 – External technical assistance needed to verify diagnoses, investigate disease, and develop response
0 – No external diagnosis or treatment resources necessary

I-5. Disease diagnoses can be made and verified rapidly

Control and treatment measures can be targeted most appropriately when the pathogen can be identified.

2 – Limited clinical diagnostics available
1 – Basic clinical and laboratory support present
0 – Advanced laboratory diagnostics available within 48 hours

I-6. Effective healthcare delivery system

Effective, accessible healthcare protects from unusual sickness and death by providing prompt disease diagnosis and treatment.

2 – Minimal availability of basic healthcare services
1 – Effective healthcare services available to those with sufficient money or prestige
0 – Effective healthcare services available to all

I-7. Healthcare delivery system able to manage highly infectious pathogens

Person-to-person transmission often occurs in hospitals when inadequate attention is paid to infection control principles.

2 – No reverse isolation patient rooms, poor observance of infection control principles
1 – Little experience with highly infectious diseases, basic infection control observed
0 – Suspect cases isolated in reverse isolation patient rooms, strong infection control practices

I-8. Effective public communication system

Effective risk communication between government agencies and the public is necessary to provide reassurance and instructions on personal steps to take to protect from disease.

2 – No effective risk communication structure or processes in place
1 – Media resources but not used regularly, entire population not reached
0 – Language-specific messages delivered by multiple media sources and messengers

I-9. Effective interagency coordination

Effective preparation and response planning requires communication and coordination among all local and central government agencies, including agriculture, veterinary medicine, public health, education, interior, communication, and security.

2 – Little regular cooperation and communication between government agencies at the central and local levels, and between these levels
1 – Interagency cooperation takes place only during a crisis and in response to pressure from senior government leaders
0 – Good interagency communication and coordination between agencies at the central government level, and between central and local authorities, as demonstrated in collaborative preparedness plans and response exercises

Total Infrastructure Factor Score: Range 0–18

Response Factors Questionnaire
(Score: 0–38)

Risk Assessment and Mitigation Factors   **Risk Score**

R-1. Authorities have identified animal reservoirs

Response efforts are more effective when animal reservoirs have been identified before the crisis occurs.

2 – Local health or public health officials are not aware of animal reservoirs
0 – Local health or public health officials are aware of animal reservoirs, or no animal reservoir exists

R-2. Authorities have identified disease transmission risk factors

Response efforts are more effective when risk factors have been considered before the crisis occurs.

2 – Local health or public health officials are not aware of disease risk factors
0 – Local health or public health officials are aware of disease risk factors

R-3. Authorities have identified high-risk groups

Response efforts are more effective when high-risk groups have been identified before the crisis occurs.

2 – Local health or public health officials are not aware of high-risk groups
0 – Local health or public health officials are aware of high-risk groups

R-4. Effective risk communication to public about disease

Early self identification of disease cases allows infectious persons to be isolated and treated.

2 – No public risk communication about disease
1 – Public announcements in mainstream media about disease symptoms, risk factors and prevention steps
0 – Comprehensive public risk communication using multiple forms of outreach about disease symptoms, risk factors, prevention steps, and where to get help and more information

R-5. Authorities have disease surveillance systems in place for animal reservoirs

Early detection and rapid response is more likely when effective surveillance systems are in place.

2 – No surveillance system in place
1 – Surveillance system implemented in response to outbreak
0 – Efficient baseline surveillance system in place

R-6. Measures (such as vaccinations when available) are in place to protect domestic animal reservoirs from diseases

Disease prevention efforts can reduce susceptibility of domestic animal populations.

2 – No preventive measures are routinely utilized
1 – Domestic animals are vaccinated when disease identified in region
0 – Domestic animals are routinely vaccinated to protect from disease

73

R-7. Measures are in place to protect domestic animal populations from wild populations

Animal-to-animal disease transmission is reduced when domestic animals are protected from exposure to diseases circulating in wild animal reservoirs.

2 – No actions are taken to protect domestic animal populations from wild animal populations
1 – Domestic animal populations are separated from wild animal populations when disease cases identified
0 – Domestic animal populations are routinely kept from contact with wild animal populations

R-8. Authorities proactively cull infected animal populations

Removal of infected animals is necessary to control animal disease spread and reduce risk of human exposure.

2 – No culling of infected animals
1 – Partial or voluntary culling of infected animal populations
0 – Institutionalized programs in place for rapid culling of infected animal populations

R-9. Authorities proactively cull exposed animal populations

Removal of exposed animals is necessary to control animal disease spread and reduce risk of human exposure.

2 – No culling of exposed animal populations
1 – Partial or voluntary culling of exposed animal populations
0 – Institutionalized programs in place for culling of exposed animal populations within 3 kilometers of diseased animals

R-10. Disease surveillance systems in place for presence of human disease

Early detection and rapid response is more likely when effective surveillance systems are in place.

2 – No surveillance system in place
1 – Surveillance system implemented in response to outbreak
0 – Efficient baseline surveillance system in place

R-11. High-risk areas are monitored for disease cases

Early detection of disease in high-risk areas may allow exposure reduction.

2 – No additional monitoring or surveillance in high-risk areas
1 – Passive detection systems used (i.e., thermal monitors in airports)
0 – Location-specific early detection procedures emphasized, i.e., authorities contact day care centers, schools, nursing homes, hospitals often to inquire about cases, provide repeated education reminders

R-12. Disease surveillance system detects pathogenicity of disease

Identification of severe versus mild cases of disease allows limited resources to be better prioritized.

2 – No surveillance system in place
1 – Surveillance system present but does not distinguish between mild and severe cases
0 – Surveillance system distinguishes mild disease cases from severe cases

R-13. Authorities perform active human case finding in vicinity of animal cases

Persons in close proximity to animals are at greater risk for exposure; actively seeking such human cases allows a faster response to new cases.

2 – No attempts to identify new disease cases in vicinity of infected animals
0 – Active human case finding started in vicinity of identified animal cases

R-14. Authorities rapidly perform contact tracing

Persons potentially exposed to infectious cases must be quickly identified and managed to interrupt disease transmission.

2 – No active contact tracing
1 – Contact tracing limited only to likely exposure groups
0 – Contact tracing identifies and contacts individuals who may have been exposed

R-15. Exposed contacts are appropriately isolated, prophylaxed, or vaccinated

Exposed persons must be treated or isolated to prevent disease transmission to others.

2 – No individual treatment of persons based on probably exposure
1 – Exposed persons are educated and instructed to seek medical attention if they develop disease symptoms
0 – Exposed persons are individually evaluated for exposure risk and are isolated, prophylaxed, or vaccinated as appropriate

R-16. Authorities appropriately isolate and treat infected persons

Active human cases must be isolated to prevent disease from being spread to others.

2 – No isolation of infected persons
1 – Voluntary or incomplete isolation during treatment
0 – Cases isolated during treatment and strong infection control in place

R-17. Disease diagnosis is rapidly made and verified

Control and treatment measures can be targeted most appropriately when the pathogen can be identified.

2 – Limited clinical diagnostics available
1 – Basic clinical and laboratory support present
0 – Advanced laboratory diagnostics available

R-18. High-quality disease treatment provided

Quality healthcare rapidly reduces disease transmission and encourages sick persons to seek treatment.

2 – Minimal availability of basic healthcare services
1 – Healthcare services available to those with sufficient money or prestige
0 – Quality healthcare services available to all

R-19. Effective interagency response coordination

An effective response requires rapid, coordinated action by all involved local and central government agencies, with little confusion about roles and responsibilities so effort is not wasted.

2 – Little evidence of coordinated crisis responses between officials at different levels of government and between government agencies
1 – Interagency cooperation occurs only during a crisis in response to pressure from senior government leaders or criticism from the media or other sources
0 – Effective coordinated interagency responses to routine emergencies and disasters

Total Response Factor Score: Range 0–38

75

Transparency Factors Questionnaire
(Score: 0–14)

Risk Assessment and Mitigation Factors   **Risk Score**

T-1. Disease containment efforts are effective

Effective disease containment measures reduce the likelihood of sustained transmission and the risk to other countries.

2 – Disease containment efforts ineffective
1 – Disease containment efforts effective only with external assistance
0 – Effective disease containment efforts

T-2. Public infrastructure maintained

Decay of basic societal services caused by (or coincidental to) disease outbreak suggests that authorities will be unable to prevent sustained transmission of disease and other countries will be at greater risk of disease introduction.

2 – Law enforcement, fire protection, healthcare services overwhelmed by disease
1 – Some interruption of essential services (water, power, telephone, food services) directly or indirectly caused by disease
0 – No interruption of public infrastructure

T-3. *Authorities openly discuss risk factors for disease, and acknowledge strengths and weaknesses in surveillance and response capabilities*

Open discussion of risk factors and system limitations implies willingness to communicate openly about disease control issues.

2 – No discussion of risk factors and system limitations in open media or official discussions
1 – Selective acknowledgement of findings when domestic or international pressure exerted or with media reporting
0 – Open discussion of risk factors, diseases, and system strengths and weaknesses

T-4. Authorities provide regular updates about disease findings within reasonable limits to protect patient privacy

Open discussion of disease outbreaks and effectiveness of interventions builds international trust and allows other countries to implement reasonable protective measures.

2 – No discussion of disease prevalence or effectiveness of control measures in open media or official discussions
1 – Selective acknowledgement of findings when domestic or international pressure exerted or with media reporting
0 – Open release of case numbers, effectiveness of disease control measures

T-5. Authorities maintain public trust

Public trust is essential for citizens to comply with instructions from authorities.

2 – Little or no evidence of public trust in government authorities, civil disorder
1 – Governmental authorities criticized in press, by other governmental authorities, and by general public
0 – Free exchange of information between public and government officials, criticism encouraged and addressed in orderly fashion

T-6. Open media reporting

Open media reporting is essential to maintaining an open society and ensuring that governmental authorities are responsive to the needs and concerns of citizens.

2 – Strict control or censorship of media reporting

1 – Limited media reporting about governmental actions

0 – Free press, open criticism of governmental authorities allowed, authorities respond to media misinformation

T-7. Open reporting to international organizations such as WHO

International organizations play important coordination and collaboration role in preventing international disease transmission.

2 – Minimal reporting to WHO, rare in-country visits permitted

1 – Reporting to WHO only in presence of international pressure

0 – Open and frequent reporting to WHO, on-site visits permitted upon request

Total Transparency Factor Score: Range 0–14

Disease-Specific Outbreak and Transmission Factors
Questionnaire
(Score: 0–36)

Risk Assessment and Mitigation Factors   **Risk Score**

DOT-1. Disease endemic in the geographic area

A disease that is continually present in an area has adapted to local environmental and biological conditions and is much more difficult to eradicate or control than one that has been recently been introduced.

2 – Disease is endemic to the area
0 – Disease is not endemic to the area

DOT-2. Disease is caused by unknown agent, or source, vehicle, or route of transmission is unusual or unknown

Lack of information about disease reservoir, transmission, and control increases risk because control measures cannot be targeted at particular areas. Extraordinarily restrictive measures are more likely to be necessary in order to control disease transmission.

2 – Agent and route of transmission are unknown
1 – Disease is understood but usual control measures are ineffective
0 – Disease and route of transmission are understood, control measures are effective

DOT-3. Disease caused by pathogen that is present in or released into the environment and has the potential to spread across international borders

Transmission could occur across political boundaries so human exposure would be greater and population movement restrictions will be less likely to control transmission.

2 – Pathogen can be carried long distances by animals, i.e., migratory waterfowl
1 – Pathogen present in or could be released into air or water
0 – Pathogen not present in the environment

DOT-4. Animal reservoir for the disease

Diseases are nearly impossible to eradicate and very difficult to control if they exist in animals.

2 – Wild animal reservoir exists
1 – Domestic animal reservoir exists
0 – No animal reservoir exists

DOT-5. Animal reservoir highly mobile

The geographic range of a disease increases if the animal reservoir freely moves around the world, while the human exposure risk increases if the animal reservoir surreptitiously follows human movement patterns (e.g., rats and plague, skunks and raccoons and rabies).

2 – Terrestrial animals adapted to manmade conveyance (i.e., truck, ship, automobile)
1 – Avian reservoir
0 – Terrestrial animal reservoir with minimal geographic range

DOT-6. Disease transmission between different types of reservoir animals

A disease is more difficult to eradicate or control if it can be transmitted from one type of animal to another, since different control measures must often be used.

2 – Disease transmission exists between types of animals (i.e., birds and pigs)
0 – No disease transmission between different types of animals

DOT-7. Mixing between susceptible wild and domestic animals

A disease that can be transmitted from wild animals to domestic animals puts these domestic animals and their human caretakers at risk for exposure.

2 – Mixing between wild and domestic animals
0 – No mixing between wild and domestic animals

DOT-8. Animal-to-human transmission of disease

Humans are at increased risk if disease can be transmitted from an animal reservoir.

2 – Easy animal-to-human transmission
1 – Rare animal-to-human transmission
0 – No animal-to-human transmission

DOT-9. Person-to-person transmission

The speed and route of person-to-person transmission has a dramatic effect on control measures.

2 – High degree of person-to-person transmission (Reproduction rate >4 (Measles =12, seasonal influenza=5))
1 – Moderate degree of person-to-person transmission (Reproduction rate 2-4 (SARS=3.5))
0 – Low degree of person-to-person transmission (Reproduction rate <2)

DOT-10. Disease pathogenicity in animal reservoir

A highly pathogenic disease that is rapidly fatal to its reservoir host is less likely to spread than a disease with few or no symptoms that allows its host to continue to move around and expose humans.

2 – Low disease pathogenicity in animal reservoir
1 – High disease pathogenicity in animal reservoir
0 – No animal reservoir or no animal-to-human transmission

DOT-11. Disease pathogenicity in humans

A highly pathogenic disease will cause more disruption to society due to sickness and death than a low pathogenic disease.

2 – High pathogenicity (>5% case fatality rate)
1 – Low pathogenicity (<4% case fatality rate)

DOT-12. Unusual disease occurrence for geographic area, season, or population

Unusual presentation may suggest a new variant of a disease or a genetically altered pathogen.

2 – Unusual or unexpected setting for disease to occur
0 – Usual disease setting

DOT-13. Evolution of cases is more severe than usual or with unusual symptoms

Unusual cases may suggest a new variant of a disease or a genetically engineered strain; usual control measures may be ineffective.

2 – Disease severity or transmission is unusually high in subgroups of people not usually highly suscept ble, i.e., young healthy adults
1 – Disease severity and transmission is unusually high in subgroups of people at increased risk, i.e., elderly, infants, immunosuppressed
0 – Normal disease severity and transmission

DOT-14. Disease occurs in area of high international traffic

Control measures are difficult to put in place across international borders without adverse economic and political consequences, so risk of widespread international transmission greatly increased.

2 – Disease transmission occurs in high traffic areas where detection and control is difficult, i.e., international airport or crowded border crossing
1 – Transmission occurs in high traffic area but surveillance systems are in place to identify and control potential cases
0 – No disease outbreaks in areas of high international traffic

DOT-15. Disease occurs in area of poor sanitation or where water- and food-borne diseases are common

Early detection and response is difficult when the background disease burden is high since new cases of a febrile disease may not become apparent until there has been person-to-person transmission.

2 – Transmission occurs in areas of high population density (>5,000 persons/km2) with poor public health infrastructure, high background disease burden
1 –Transmission occurs in areas (<5000 persons/km2) with poor public health infrastructure, high background disease burden
0 – No disease exists in areas with high background disease burdens

DOT-16. Increased mobility of high-risk groups exists

High-risk agricultural and healthcare workers may be the principle sources of spread of a highly infectious disease.

2 – High risk groups come into contact with many other people in the course of their usual activities (i.e., healthcare workers who live in an urban area; agricultural workers who travel to markets)
0 – No particular increased exposure risk of high-risk groups

DOT-17. Disease cases develop among healthcare personnel

Excessive sickness and death among healthcare delivery personnel could rapidly degrade healthcare system.

2 – Disease occurs in healthcare personnel despite usual infection control measures
1 – Rare disease cases occur in healthcare personnel
0 – No disease cases occur in healthcare personnel

DOT-18. Initial disease case (Index case) has high-risk travel or exposure history

Increases risk of rapid international spread of pathogens that are not usually anticipated by healthcare personnel and so are more likely to be misdiagnosed.

2 – Index case recently traveled to region with exposure risk
1 – Index case in close proximity to potentially infectious cases, i.e., international traveler or highly mobile population
0 – No unusual travel or exposure

Total Disease Specific Outbreak and Transmission Factor Score: Range 0–36

Appendix B
Risk Assessment and Mitigation Factors Worksheets

- *Ecological Factors*

- *Infrastructure Factors*

- *Response Factors*

- *Transparency Factors*

- *Disease-Specific Outbreak and Transmission Factors*

- *Post-Assessment*

84

Step 1: Local Self-Assessment

ECOLOGICAL FACTORS WORKSHEET

(Choices and corresponding scores for Ecological Factors E-1 through E-6 are explained in Appendix A)

Factor	Score	Description
E-1		
E-2		
E-3		
E-4		
E-5		
E-6		
TOTAL Ecological Factors Score:		

INFRASTRUCTURE FACTORS WORKSHEET

(Choices and corresponding scores for Infrastructure Factors I-1 through I-9 are explained in Appendix A)

Factor	Score	Description
I-1		
I-2		
I-3		
I-4		
I-5		
I-6		
I-7		
I-8		
I-9		
TOTAL Infrastructure Factors Score:		

Step 1: Local Self-Assessment

RESPONSE FACTORS WORKSHEET

(Choices and corresponding scores for Response Factors R-1 through R-19 are explained in Appendix A)

Factor	Score	Description
R-1		
R-2		
R-3		
R-4		
R-5		
R-6		
R-7		
R-8		
R-9		
R-10		
R-11		
R-12		
R-13		
R-14		
R-15		
R-16		
R-17		
R-18		
R-19		
TOTAL Response Factors Score:		

Step 2: External Perceptions

TRANSPARENCY FACTORS WORKSHEET

(Choices and corresponding scores for Transparency Factors T-1 through T-7 are explained in Appendix A)

Factor	Score	Description
T-1		
T-2		
T-3		
T-4		
T-5		
T-6		
T-7		
TOTAL Transparency Factors Score:		

DISEASE-SPECIFIC OUTBREAK AND TRANSMISSION (DOT) FACTORS

(Choices and corresponding scores for DOT Factors DOT-1 through DOT-18 are explained in Appendix A)

Factor	Description	WHO Phases[60]					
		1	2	3	4	5	6
DOT-1							
DOT-2							
DOT-3							
DOT-4							
DOT-5							
DOT-6							
DOT-7							
DOT-8							
DOT-9							
DOT-10							
DOT-11							
DOT-12							
DOT-13							
DOT-14							
DOT-15							
DOT-16							
DOT-17							
DOT-18							
TOTAL Disease Outbreak and Transmission Factors Scores							

[60] WHO phases are described on page 39 in Summary of WHO Global Pandemic Phases.

POST-ASSESSMENT WORKSHEET

FACTOR	SCORE		COMMENT
	Pre-	Post-	
Ecological Factors—No change poss ble			
Infrastructure Factors—Decrease from _____ to _____			
I-1			
I-2			
I-3			
I-4			
I-5			
I-6			
I-7			
I-8			
I-9			
Response Factors—Decrease from _____ to _____			
R-1			
R-2			
R-3			
R-4			
R-5			
R-6			
R-7			
R-8			
R-9			
R-10			

R-11			
R-12			
R-13			
R-14			
R-15			
R-16			
R-17			
R-18			
R-19			

Transparency Factors—Decrease from _____ to _____

T-1			
T-2			
T-3			
T-4			
T-5			
T-6			
T-7			

Post-Intervention Self-Assessment Results	Pre-	Post-
Local Baseline Risk (LBR)		
International Baseline Risk (IBR)		
International Response Posture (WHO Pandemic Phase 3)		

TOTAL SCORES GUIDE: LOW=<50   MODERATE=51-100   HIGH=>100

91

www.ingramcontent.com/pod-product-compliance
Lightning Source LLC
Chambersburg PA
CBHW081549170526
45166CB00009B/2626